'Christine's insider account of dementia, focusing on the continuing sense of self in the disease, brings a powerful message of hope for people who have dementia, their families and health care providers. People with dementia are still people of worth, even in the face of increasing cognitive decline and memory dysfunction.'

– Rev Prof Elizabeth MacKinlay, CAPS, Australian Centre for Christianity and Culture, St Mark's National Theological Centre and School of Theology, Charles Stuart University

'Christine Bryden demonstrates powerfully that, despite dementia, her self and desire to improve her community are intact, that people living with dementia can enjoy mutually positive relationships with others and that we honor our own humanity ever more deeply when we honor the humanity of people living with dementia.'

– Steven R. Sabat, PhD, Professor Emeritus of Psychology, Georgetown University, Washington, DC, USA

'The question of what makes "me" me and how I can hold on to my sense of self in the midst of the challenges of dementia is to say the least, challenging. What is it that holds me in my selfhood and identity when I seem to be forgetting all of the old markers that held me in place? Christine Bryden offers a profound challenge to such false assumptions. Through narrative, personal reflection and enlightening philosophical reflection, Christine opens up fresh space for hope within which the complex cadences of personal and communal selfhood can be understood in ways that enable people truly to live with dementia.'

– Rev Prof John Swinton, Professor in Practical Theology and Pastoral Care, King's College, University of Aberdeen

'Christine Bryden is a remarkable woman, and a pioneering dementia advocate, one I am proud to call a friend. *Will I Still Be Me?* is a tribute to her continued commitment to improve the lives of all people with dementia, which gives us hope, and deep insight into how her spirituality has supported her to live positively with dementia. Christine has given the world another great gift; her writing, her research and her appraisal of an insider's view of how dementia affects so much more than one individual.'

– Kate Swaffer, human rights activist and author of What the Hell Happened to My Brain?

WILL I STILL BE ME?

WILL I STILL BE ME?

Finding a Continuing Sense of Self in the Lived Experience of Dementia

CHRISTINE BRYDEN

Jessica Kingsley *Publishers*
London and Philadelphia

First published in 2018
by Jessica Kingsley Publishers
73 Collier Street
London N1 9BE, UK
and
400 Market Street, Suite 400
Philadelphia, PA 19106, USA

www.jkp.com

Library of Congress Cataloging in Publication Data
Names: Bryden, Christine, 1949- author.
Title: Will I still be me? : finding a continuing sense of self in the lived experience of dementia / Christine Bryden.
Description: London ; Philadelphia : Jessica Kingsley Publishers, 2018. | Includes bibliographical references and index.
Identifiers: LCCN 2018002347 | ISBN 9781785925559 (alk. paper)
Subjects: LCSH: Bryden, Christine, 1949---Mental health. | Dementia--Patients--Biography. | Alzheimer's disease--Patients--Biography.
Classification: LCC RC523.3 .B796 2018 | DDC 616.8/310092 [B] --dc23

British Library Cataloguing in Publication Data
A CIP catalogue record for this book is available from the British Library

ISBN 978 1 78592 555 9
eISBN 978 1 78450 950 7

Printed and bound in Great Britain

Contents

Acknowledgements

This book is drawn from secular aspects of my thesis for a PhD, which was supported by a Public and Contextual Theology Research Centre Scholarship from the Charles Sturt University School of Theology, St Mark's National Theological Centre. My PhD supervisors – Professor Elizabeth MacKinlay and Dr Jane Foulcher – provided invaluable advice and guidance. Paul Bryden gave very helpful sub-editorial assistance.

I am very thankful for the insights of the many people with dementia who I have met over the years, whose stories are reflected in the vignettes introducing the various sections of the book.

Jessica Kingsley and her wonderful staff have been very supportive of me over the years, and I am particularly grateful to their enthusiastic response to my thesis outline, as well as to the final document. Jessica Kingsley Publishers have a significant list of books that reach out and support people with dementia and their families, and I am humbled to be one of their authors.

Preface

I was diagnosed with dementia in 1995, over 20 years ago now. I have easily outlasted all predictions made for my prognosis, and indeed any loss of self, and I still feel very much 'me'. As I often say, 'I'm still here!' I have come to see that the outsider's view of loss of self is unhelpful, and does not reflect the true insider's experience of those of us living with dementia. I can bear witness to my own experience of restoring my life after a traumatic diagnosis, as well as attesting to the many stories of others who are living with dementia and continue to live their lives full of meaning.

I have used vignettes to introduce the various sections of the book, which are based on the experiences of many of the people living with dementia who I have met over the years. I have changed all names and removed any identifying material, in order to ensure their privacy. I have also conflated some of the experiences that have been shared with me, in order to cover the gamut of these experiences, but nonetheless the resulting pictures are a valid representation of a whole range of perspectives on living with dementia.

I hope that this book will help society to see people with dementia, like myself, with new eyes, and realise that there is in fact no loss of self in dementia, although our cognitive self is indeed changing and altering our experiences of the world. The idea of loss of self in dementia is oppressive and leads to an overwhelming fear, but what is the proof? Up until now, all we have had are the opinions of *outside* observers; no one living with dementia has described this concept from the *insider*'s view. I want to challenge this story of total loss of all aspects of self in dementia: we are not disappearing, nor are we dying in small steps, and our families are not losing us bit by bit. We are fully present, even though we are gradually interacting with, and experiencing, the world differently.

I suggest that three aspects of our sense of self continue throughout the lived experience of dementia:

Embodied self: my sense of being embodied as an 'I' with first-person feelings about the world around me, able to distinguish self from non-self.

Relational self: my sense of being an embodied self in relationships with others and with what gives me a sense of meaning.

Narrative self: my sense of being able to find meaning in life and develop a sense of identity in the present moment.

My aim is to encourage society to look beyond the dominant story of loss of self in dementia, so that people with all varying cognitive and physical capacities can be included and welcomed as equals. I seek in particular to transform society's views, towards accepting that there is a continuing sense of self throughout the lived experience of dementia, so that people with dementia and their families can be better supported in inclusive and diverse communities. I look to a future in which people with dementia are included as equals within such communities, rather than being regarded as defective autonomous individuals.

In a diverse community, people of all varying physical and cognitive capacities, who have difficulties in today's fast-paced world, can be included as equals, where what is important is who we are, not what we do. *We are all human beings, not human doings.* This is good news for all those of us living with dementia, as we are who we are.

In a community that emphasises diversity and equality, we can feel welcomed and as if we belong, despite our communication problems and recall difficulties. Others can come alongside us in our present moment, carrying our story, and thereby challenging the story of loss. We might need help in finding meaning and nourishing our spirit, but we are still fully present alongside others in this community. Highlighting what remains in dementia, my aim is to encourage society to see people living with dementia with new eyes.

Christine Bryden PhD
Person living with dementia, advocate and author
Adjunct Research Fellow, Public and Contextual Theology
Research Centre, Charles Sturt University Australia
February 2018

1

Am I Losing My Self?

The journey of becoming, of leaving behind previous perceptions of who we are, is common to us all, as part of our life's narrative. We discover new aspects of our selves as time goes by. Yet those of us diagnosed with dementia fear a very different journey – one of loss, of losing our relationships, not only with others, but with what gives us meaning in life. We wonder if and when we will experience a future loss of self. My diagnosis with dementia was in 1995, and I have published several works since that time, reflecting on the lived experience with an insider's view (Bryden 2002, 2005, 2012, 2015a, 2015b, 2016; Bryden and MacKinlay 2002). These publications were aimed at providing an alternative view to the dominant story of dementia through the lens of my lived experience. They tracked my changing sense of self, challenged the common perceptions of dementia, and highlighted some of my fears of future loss.

In this book I explore in much more detail the key issue emerging from this body of work, which is the supposed loss of self in dementia. This idea that we might lose our self due to dementia overwhelms us at the time of diagnosis, and we feel oppressed by the surrounding views of society that this is what faces us now, or at some time in the future. For example, it is common to hear such offhand comments as, 'She's no longer there' or 'He is slipping away to dementia', which demonstrate the usual view of dementia as being accompanied by a loss of self. This view of loss of self has an extremely negative impact on those of us being diagnosed with dementia, and cannot be underestimated. Facing a possible future loss of self results in a paralysing fear, which I expressed in the title of my first book, *Who Will I Be When I Die?* (Bryden 1998, rev. 2012). This was written shortly after my diagnosis, when I felt extremely fearful of the future, and withdrew from social contact due to such negative views.

In this book, I am looking at dementia from the inside out, using narrative as 'a crucial conceptual category for... depicting personal identity' (Hauerwas and Jones 1989, p.5), revealing the self in its indivisible unity of body and mind (Crites 1971, p.85). Narrative is a 'qualitative or interpretative research method...[in which] researchers study things in their natural settings, attempting to make sense of and interpret phenomena in terms of the meaning people bring to them' (Moen 2006, p.61). It is very useful for exploring a continuing sense of self within the lived experience of dementia, searching for meaning from within the setting, in order to transform the understanding of 'that experience for [myself] and others' (Clandinin and Roziek 2006, p.42).

I examine my inner history of self, which gives a very different perspective to 'the outer history of things' (Neibuhr 1941, pp.33, 30). From this inner perspective, I describe my disturbed sense of time, rather than an accurate awareness of chronological time; therefore my narrative is not based on precise facts, but on a subjective search for meaning. It builds on my existing body of work in a 'continuously developing narrative that is constantly forming and changing form' (Moen 2006, p.60), aiming to give an insider's perspective of a sense of self in dementia, and continuing to challenge the dominant story of loss.

Writing a book is not at all easy at the best of times, and now there are extensive challenges due to my dementia. These make the process of writing and analysis more difficult, yet at the same time more authentic, because my increasing impairment gives insight into my sense of self from within the lived experience. I live with dementia and can reflect both about, and from within, my difficulties and fears in order to delve deeper into meaning. Impairment has invaded my present moment in what feels like a folded sense of time, so I am continually reminded of loss. This can even be seen in my various publications, in which there is a conflict of tenses between being and becoming, and loss and gain. I have attempted to counter the discourses of loss with an alternative story, yet on occasion I keep returning to a story of impairment. I feel drawn downwards into the spiral of the usual negative view of dementia resulting in a loss of self, even as I try to write about my own experiences in order to challenge this view.

I continue to experience a tension between my sense of a coherent self, and a fear of a possible future loss of self; on occasion, I am still negatively impacted by the dominant story of dementia. The potential loss of self looms large, despite my focus on challenging this from my own insider's perspective. Although diagnosis impacted upon my concept of meaning in life, I began to resolve my fears and feelings through my published work, even as I skirted around my central concern of loss of self. My continuing difficulties now provide an authentic basis for my reflections on this key issue in this book.

Despite cognitive impairment, I have been able to examine my published work, refer to relevant literature, and reflect on the meaning of my ongoing experience in the present moment. This has taken an immense amount of effort: making many notes about what I am reading, so that I can find references once again on my computer, and also extensive note taking – even in the middle of the night – about any ideas that come to me. Yet despite the effort that this takes, I can give an authentic experiential account of dementia from an insider's perspective, which provides alternative insights into the idea of loss of self. I explore a continuing sense of self, in embodied relationships within the community, where I retain the ability to find a sense of meaning in the present moment. My aim has been, and continues to be, to project a new world of possibility and to 'redescribe reality', so that people with dementia can be seen in a very different way (Fiddes 2000, p.38).

2

Re-interpreted and Re-packaged at Diagnosis!

Tom and his wife Mary sat in the specialist's rooms, anxiously waiting for a diagnosis. Tom had been having some problems with remembering things and getting words right for some time now. Even keeping score at his regular golf games with his group of friends was becoming increasingly difficult. So their usual doctor had sent him off to a specialist for a whole series of tests – recalling shopping lists, words, drawing pictures, clocks, as well as noisy brain scans. Tom and Mary were now in the specialist's rooms, waiting for the results. The specialist looked up from Tom's notes, and said, 'I'm afraid that there are clear signs of dementia. There is no other reason for all of these problems, and little that can be done to help. I suggest that you both go home and get Tom's affairs in order.' Mary felt frozen to the spot – would this mean that she would lose Tom to dementia? Would he become nothing more than an empty shell of a body?

Tom was in total shock. He had heard so much that was negative about dementia, and felt that he really couldn't face this fearful future. Surely, just before going into the specialist's rooms, he had been quite normal? Now, just an hour later, he had this terrifying and devastating label attached to him. What would his friends think of him? Would they still be his friends? Mary was in tears; surely she was not going to lose her husband to this awful dementia? They were both disbelieving at Tom's sudden transformation into nothing but a person with dementia.

At the age of 46, I was a high-level career civil servant, advising the Australian prime minister on science and technology. How long ago that seems now – ancient history maybe? I certainly cannot feel any real connection with this science and technology advisor, who seems more like a long lost friend than me! For a few years or so, I had been struggling with extreme and frequent headaches, as well as confusion, including problems with words and finding my way. I thought these were all signs of stress, as I certainly had a very demanding job and was finding that life as a recently divorced mother of three girls, aged 9, 13 and 19, increasingly difficult to juggle. The youngest two were at home with me, and the eldest had just moved away to go to university.

At last I found the time to go to a doctor, who was quite concerned, and she referred me for brain scans and tests to check what might be going on. It was a nice break from work to lie on the scanning table, and I tried hard to ignore the reality of what might be found. But rather than any tumour, the scans showed a significant loss of brain, and the testing showed that I was also having a range of thinking difficulties. This seemed to alarm the doctor, who referred me straightaway to a specialist. He bluntly told me that I had probable dementia and should retire from work immediately – indeed, that very week – and should not be in any position of responsibility (Bryden 2012). This was a devastating diagnosis at the age of only 46 – surely dementia only happened to much older people? The diagnosis was extremely traumatic, as I had only just obtained my divorce from an abusive first husband (Bryden 2012, 2015a) and was about to move to a new house with my two youngest daughters. My eldest daughter took time off to help us – these were such terrible times!

Hanging over me were the roiling and ominous black clouds of the loss of self that was supposed to occur with dementia. Would I know my daughters? Would I even know myself? Who would I be when I died? The specialist told me that it would be a few years till I was in full-time care, and then only a few years more until I died. This would be in my early 50s, so I believed that I would miss out on my daughters' teenage years, weddings, births, and their future. They too would miss out on having their mother one day soon. I felt paralysed with a fear of loss for my daughters, and fears of the terrible picture that I had of dying with dementia. But now it has been over 20 years since that awful time, and *I am still here*, showing that these prognoses and fears were wrong. No, I am not living in some 'make-believe' land, and I struggle to cope most days, finding language, way-finding and recall increasingly problematic. I am indeed declining steadily, but now have a wonderful husband by my side to help me (see Bryden 2005).

Diagnosis had disrupted my story of a future high-level career reliant on continued cognitive function. It confronted me with the dominant *biomedical* story of dementia, which is that increasing brain damage leads to loss of all faculties. I felt oppressed by the power of the prognosis that I would gradually lose my sense of self, as my brain continued to atrophy; it was as if my story had become 're-interpreted, re-packaged, and re-presented... to conform to the objective and scientific basis of medicine' (Clark 2001, p.195). When I looked to the *psychosocial* description of dementia, this also gave me little hope, as it discussed how I would become increasingly dependent on others to relate to me throughout my lived experience of dementia, when presumably I would decline and lose my sense of self. Just like the biomedical view, I felt that I was little more than this dementia, setting me apart from society. I would be nothing but a physical body, relying on others for my sense of self.

As an important part of this psychosocial view, the psycho-gerontologist, Tom Kitwood, introduced the term *personhood* to describe the relationship with our family and friends, who bestow this sense of self on us (1997, p.8). But what if they were to die or no longer visit, and paid helpers cared only for my physical needs? In that case, surely I would become devoid of personhood, and perhaps indeed only be a physical body? Philosopher Stephen Ames highlights this risk: 'Defining "personhood" as an attributed status makes personhood vulnerable as a status to be withheld [if] the person is not recognized, indeed not recognizable' (2016, p.127). Bestowal of personhood implies a one-way relationship, in which the others actively bestow some capacities and attributes to the person with dementia, who passively receives these. The idea comes from outside observation of people with dementia and their interactions with care-partners.

At this point, I want to emphasise my use of the term *care-partner*, which I first began to use in my talks during 2003 to highlight how we need not be only the passive recipient of care, but can also be active contributors towards expressing our needs in a caring partnership with others. The word carer or caregiver implies that there is a one-way giving of care by others to us, whereby we are the passive recipients of that care. I wanted to give this relationship a new perspective, of giving and receiving in an equal partnership, where I express my needs as a care-partner. This caring relationship can involve the person with dementia, their families, paid helpers, as well as friends – all participating in a caring partnership. By 2012, I started also to use the term *enabler* as an even more positive term: my husband helps me to keep on doing as much as I can, while I can. He enables me, which feels liberating, as it allows me to focus on continuing those activities that I still feel able to do, while my husband takes on more and more other activities to help me.

In my published work, I have criticised the biomedical view (Bryden 2015b, p.28), which describes an increasing loss of cognitive ability, leading to the idea of a loss of self.

The psychosocial discourse similarly focuses on loss and the need for the bestowal of personhood by care-partners. Neither viewpoint takes into account the impact of increasing difficulties in my daily life, nor how I experience the world around me, despite and with my dementia. They speak *for me and about me*, rather than letting me express verbally or nonverbally how I feel my impairment daily. Both of these outsiders' views focus on loss of personhood. In contrast, I am writing from an insider's perspective, so I choose to use the term *self*, as expressed by first-person language and defined in the social constructionist literature as the 'self of personal identity' (Sabat 2001, p.17). Rather than personhood, *self* expresses how I have a mental representation of myself as the centre of my conscious agency, necessary for me to relate to others, and to think about thinking, deciding and doing (Brown 1998, p.108). This is not dependent on any act of others, and demonstrates how I have a mental feeling of 'I' as a continuous whole throughout my life, which is making sense of the world over time.

I am experiencing the world differently along this journey with dementia, as my cognition declines, but who am I as a physical, emotional and spiritual being examining various aspects of my self in this context? Although I have related to the world differently since my diagnosis, still my subjective sense of self remains, perceiving and interacting with my changing material, social and spiritual environments. I am not simply a bundle of attributes, or a certain personality; there is much more to my life, my relationships and my sense of unity, which is shaping my personal identity (Bryan 2016, p.13). I am far more than a deteriorating self in an increasingly empty shell of a body, with disappearing neurones and neuronal pathways.

3

How Can I Write a Book?

Helen had only just been diagnosed with dementia, and was in total shock. What would be ahead for her? As an avid writer of personal journals, she thought it would be a great idea to write down her thoughts and feelings, to share with her family and friends over time. But how could she possibly carry on doing this, given that the doctor had told her she might not be able to write any more by the end of the year in six months, and that she should quickly get her affairs in order? He had said that she might not even be able to sign her own name by the end of the year. Was it even worth starting to write things down? Her thoughts were muddled and, when she wrote, the letters kept on coming out peculiarly shaped. Her friend, Jane, listened to her fears of the future, and did not respond by saying 'No that will never happen'. Jane understood that these were very real fears that needed to be heard, and encouraged Helen, saying that she would be happy to help her at any stage. Even if Helen could no longer write, Jane would ask her questions and write down her thoughts. Jane said this was a journey that was so important, far too important to be left just between them, and that she might even try to find someone to publish it all eventually. Wow! This was overwhelming for Helen, who was amazed that her ideas might be that important to anyone, but she loved writing and sharing, so agreed this could be a journey they could begin together – even if she might not make it until the end.

During the months of tests and scans following my referral to the specialist, and leading up to my confirmed diagnosis, I met Reverend Professor Elizabeth MacKinlay, and realising that she was both a gerontologist and priest, I asked her to journey with me into my unknown future (see Bryden 2012, Foreword). We became the 'storyteller and the story listener', as we explored my fears of a future journey with dementia (MacKinlay 2016, p.29). My question was: 'Is it possible to find meaning in dementia?' (MacKinlay 2016, p.26). I wanted to find meaning during this terrible time of testing, and the possible diagnosis of dementia, including re-examining my perceptions of self, brain and mind.

I shared with Liz my feelings and fears, and quietly she listened, reflected, and was able to put my fears in perspective. She never dismissed any of my fears of the future, but was able to help me work my way through them. Liz strongly encouraged me to write these views down, as she had never spoken with a person with dementia, only nursed them in the later stages. The voice of a person with dementia was so very new, so unexpected, and might well 'upset the applecart' of all those experts who had been talking about dementia from the outside observation of their patients. Liz was discovering from me how the idea of loss impacted on the feelings of the person being given the diagnosis of dementia; she was learning about the unseen internal struggles that we had in coping with the views of society around us, let alone the views within us, in response to our own beliefs in this terrible concept.

I began to write about my lived experience of dementia, although I did not focus solely on this key theme of loss of self in dementia (Bryden 2002, 2005, 2012, 2015a, 2015b, 2016; Bryden and MacKinlay 2002) as it was too overwhelming, particularly when I first started writing in 1998. Apart from anything else, writing as a person living with dementia was a very new concept at that time: I was challenging all those biomedical and psychosocial experts, and it was a struggle even to be believed. Surely I did not have dementia if I could write? Surely the diagnosis was wrong? So I described my journey more as a series of events, and my reactions to them, rather than examining in detail the fear of losing my self, whilst being surrounded by the usual view of dementia.

In this book I seek to delve further into these struggles with my own fears of a loss of self in dementia. I challenge the outsider's perception by looking at my own experiences, as well as at some relevant literature, in order to provide an integrating insider's view. The method I use is called autoethnography: I analyse (graphy) my own subjective lived experience (auto), in order to shed light on a continuing sense of self throughout dementia (ethno). I am analysing the concept of loss of self from the perspective of a cultural group of which I am a member (people living with dementia), so have complete member researcher status (Ellis and Bochner 2000) and can provide an insider's perspective.

My book is an *evocative* form of autoethnography, which is described as a way 'to change the world by writing from the heart' (Denzin 2006, p.422). I hope to prompt society to see people with dementia through different eyes, by exposing my vulnerable self, where this shows that I am 'trying to preserve or restore the continuity and coherence of life's unity in the face of unexpected blows of fate' (Ellis and Bochner 2000, p.744). This quote goes to the heart of my efforts to challenge the common view of loss of self, and how outsiders' perspectives of dementia threatened the continuity and coherence of my life's unity in the face of my diagnosis.

Surely an insider's voice is far more authentic than that of an independent researcher (Wall 2015, p.153), because I am inside what I am studying? I am looking at how my experience has meaning and 'by exploring a particular life, I hope to understand a way of life' (Ellis and Bochner 2000, p.737). How could someone who does not have dementia explore the sense of self within the lived experience? However, I am also 'both an insider and an outsider' (Baker 2001, p.399), as I once lived without a diagnosis and believed the usual view of loss of self in dementia. It was this belief in future loss of self that made the diagnosis more traumatic, as I feared that I would indeed experience this at some time. Importantly, therefore, I am not only a complete member researcher, but also once shared an outsider's perspective of dementia. I can look at loss of self in dementia from both points of view.

How can I overcome cognitive difficulties?

A former English teacher, Doug had been diagnosed a year or so ago now, and was really struggling to keep track of time, recall things and speak properly. Yet vocabulary was once his greatest strength. He tried to tell his wife, Marge, about it, but often he could only come out with jumbled words and muddled grammar. Marge just couldn't understand how bad it was for him to feel like this, and always made light of it, saying it was just a bit of memory loss. Maybe she was trying to make him feel better? But for Doug, the weeks seemed to slip by, and somehow even felt lumpy; it was almost as if today and last week oscillated between the present and the past. He was always pacing the house, trying to remember why he had gone from one room to another – it felt exhausting. The only time he really could forget everything and simply enjoy life was when he slipped on his headphones, took out a new CD, and began to listen. Doug could forget all his problems and be taken up into the beauty of his music, absorbed and uplifted. He felt like himself again, with no problems to worry about. These beautiful new pieces of classical music made his spirits soar, so that everything seemed to fade totally into the background. He couldn't understand why people only listened to old music written centuries ago, when there was so much being written every year by a whole range of modern composers. It would be like reading Austen or Dickens over and over again! But when he was without his music and needed to go about his ordinary life from day to day, Doug felt adrift somehow, lost without an anchor. He couldn't recall what he did yesterday, or even what day it was today, let alone what he had done in the last few weeks, and so felt very lost. What turmoil he lived in, and even his wonderful wife had no idea what it was like! Recall of events, names and places were all slippery, so that it was like trying to grab an idea as it floated past, but it was too soon far out of reach and totally forgotten. Doug felt as if his recall for things was disappearing into a deep black hole, beyond his grasp. He'd be thinking of something to say, turn to Marge to share this thought; his mouth would open and there would be no word, let alone a thought, and all he could do was mutter about having forgotten yet again. It was all becoming so very frustrating! Even worse was that, even if Doug did remember a word, he could not always pronounce it properly. He felt as if words were disappearing, being flung out like the countless stars into the vast and infinite universe, way beyond his reach.

Before diagnosis, I had an anticipation of my future, as well as knowledge of my past, so I felt firmly planted on a timeline, but now my sense of time is impaired. I feel as if there is an ever-changing flux of the present moment, where time passing has become like a flickering light, illuminating fragmented and disconnected landmarks in my life. I can relate to the feelings of the character in the novel *The Forgotten*: 'Time no longer flowed, but toppled over the edge of a yawning precipice ... He was losing sight of his landmarks' (Wiesel 1992, p.262). Despite a confusing and shifting parade of scenes in my past and into the future, I am aware of the present moment, or what neuropsychologist Steven Sabat calls the 'personal present' (Sabat 2001, p.232). I have this intense sense of this moment, but the fear of loss of self in dementia, as well as my increasing impairment, 'haunt[s] the present' (Frank 2013, p.60). This invasion of negative feelings into my present moment feels like a dark cloud of despair hanging over me, which I keep needing to escape. I have increasing difficulties with recall of yesterday, last week, or what I plan tomorrow or next week, so that I feel as if I have lost track of where I am on a timeline (Bryden 2015b, p.97). Again, I can relate to the character in *The Forgotten*, who reflects, 'But what is man deprived of memory? Not even a shadow... I'd have preferred death to this agony of memories wrestling and drowning' (Wiesel 1992, p.313).

My lack of recall is not memory loss, as my memories lurk around just out of reach, so that with prompts I can be helped to find these in the quicksand of my dysfunctional brain. I find that by using the calendar application on my phone, computer and tablet, I have a timeline once more, a reference for trying to reconstruct my life as it flows from one week to the next. I refer to my problem as *recall dysfunction*, which is not a lack of memory for facts about my past, as with help I can access feelings, meaning and my flow of awareness within the lived experience of dementia. Despite needing this help, I can still focus on the meaning in the present moment, and can give an insider's viewpoint to what it feels like to have these challenges.

Another major challenge in my reflective writing, as well as in my speaking, is a decreasing vocabulary and grammar. There is no thesaurus that will help me find the word or phrase that has become elusive, as all I have left are vague concepts, so cannot search for the synonyms or antonyms. In my head 'a string of pictures has formed, but the words for those pictures no longer make their way into [my] consciousness' (Bryden 2005, p.118). Athough I rarely find the words or sentence structure for which I am searching, nonetheless I can still reflect on meaning. However, writing now takes an increasing length of time and effort, and of course spelling and grammar check on the computer are essential!

How can I find meaning?

Neil had been struggling to cope with having dementia for some time now – he wasn't sure for quite how long. He couldn't remember names; from time to time he would even struggle to recall his dear wife, Fay's, name. It wasn't that he didn't know Fay, but that her name just seemed to escape somewhere. Labels for people were increasingly hard to attach! His struggles would sometimes overwhelm him and lead to an outburst of frustration, when he would yell out, because nothing was making sense and everything was simply too hard and stressful. He felt like a pressure cooker, where the steam was building up uncontrollably due to all this stress. At the end of each day, Fay would gently suggest that he should take their old dog, Misty, for a walk down to the nearby park. This was a wonderful time of peace for Neil, when he and Misty would potter along, looking at the various plants, listening to the different birds, and seeing the sky high above with its ever-changing cloud patterns. He would appreciate the passing seasons, except of course the heat of summer that made it hard to go for much of a walk. Neil's favourite thing was to take some duck food down to the lake, where there were a few white ducks and a goose, which would come waddling and quacking to meet him each day. These daily walks were a simple pleasure that eased away the stress and made him almost forget he had dementia: they gave him an inner sense of peace. Sometimes Fay would go with him, but mostly she would just make sure that Neil took a phone with him, so that she could check up, just in case he felt lost.

My sense of time, recall and language are gradually becoming more impaired, yet I can still explore my continuing sense of self. I grapple for words just out of reach; I struggle with many daily tasks (Bryden 2015a, pp.215–229), but I am still Christine, who can search for meaning within her lived experience of dementia. My cognition is indeed deteriorating, but I can explore my experience in the present moment, and reflect on my unfolding narrative to discover a continuing sense of self, within my changing experiences of and interactions with the world.

The fear of a future loss of self that faced me after diagnosis prompted my published work, in which I examine a few issues in the context of their meaning, and describe events in my life. Now, several years on, I examine the integrating theme of loss, delving further into its meaning, recognising that 'Often a seeming tragedy can lead us to great spiritual insight and personal transformation' (Grudzen and Oberle 2001, p.182). With the fading of my factual story, a narrative approach to wisdom has helped me, where wisdom is 'the acceptance of our lifestory; as it is, as it has been, and also as it has not been – "the road not chosen"' (Kenyon and Randall 2001, p.10). I have finally been able to accept my new life with dementia, and do as much as I can, while I can, to reach out and help others by speaking and writing about what I am learning along the way.

At the beginning after diagnosis, I was overcome with feelings of anxiety at a potential future loss of self, and needed to uncover 'the strength of the spiritual dimension within' (Kuhl and Westwood 2001, p.322). However, since that time I have been greatly reassured by reading that spirituality does not need cognition or language (MacKinlay 2011, p.43). I have found meaning by turning to my Christian faith, where at 'the heart of…Christian spirituality is God's approach to human beings' (Swinton 2012, p.174). I did not have to earn my way to God somehow, and could simply allow God to reach out to me in my pain and confusion. Indeed, I experienced a sense of transcendence, where this is described as moving 'beyond self-centredness to other-centredness' (MacKinlay and Trevitt 2012, p.86). For me, I became more other-centred through advocacy for people with dementia and their families, which became central to giving me a sense of meaning and purpose in life.

Why the idea of loss of self impacted negatively on me

Seiji was a high-flying sales executive with a major company, and was experiencing a few problems with memory, numbers and words. He thought nothing of it, dismissing this all as stress. He worked very long hours and his job was demanding, involving lots of travel, a big group reporting to him and a boss who seemed to ask more of him each time he had accomplished something. Being a top sales person was who he was, central to his sense of identity. Seiji still felt successful, despite this stress, but when he took a few days off, and these little problems did not seem to go away, he began to feel more concerned. He talked to his wife, Emi, who said she had noticed he was getting a bit absent-minded, but surely this was nothing much to worry about? However, when he got back after his short break, Seiji was called in to see the boss, who said that he had made some important mistakes recently. There were some problems with Seiji's billing calculations, as well as him using the wrong names for some important clients, and mixing up a few customer orders. Also, one of the staff had noted that Seiji had not recalled an important decision made at a recent meeting. The boss asked if there was anything he should know about, and that perhaps Seiji should go for a medical check-up just in case. The doctor seemed quite concerned to hear what had been going on at work, and referred

Seiji to a neurologist. What a palaver then ensued, as Seiji had to go for tests and brain scans, taking time off work when he really needed to be there – he had never taken time off during annual sales report and review time, which was a critical time of year! Seiji and Emi were then both called back to see the specialist, and were absolutely devastated to hear that Seiji was showing the early signs of dementia. How could this be? This was so shameful: how could Seiji possibly tell his boss, his colleagues or his staff? The boss was incredulous, and said he would never have suspected it, recommending that Seiji take a few months off work, until 'things sorted themselves out'. The main problem for Seiji was emotional: he felt absolutely devastated, as his intellect had been the driving force behind his successful career, and he still felt very capable. Who was he, if he was not a top sales person? Who was he, if he no longer went to work? How could he possibly have this condition of old age in his 50s, and how could he possibly face a future loss of who he was?

Some underlying assumptions about the importance of intellect and what it means to be a 'self' influenced me profoundly after my diagnosis with dementia. The negative impact of the diagnosis drove me to examine what might continue through the lived experience of dementia, and what this could mean for the community. Up until the time of my diagnosis with dementia, I regarded my fully functioning brain as a key aspect of my self. 'Being highly intelligent was so much a part of who I was. My brain was my identity' (Bryden 2015a, p.139). I was a task-oriented decision-maker at work, and at home, and saw the world through the lens of my intellect. How could I possibly cope with losing my brain over time, as surely that would mean losing who I was?

But in 1990, I had a Christian conversion experience: 'I felt filled to overflowing with joy and peace' (Bryden 2012, p.132). I experienced emotional and spiritual aspects of my sense of self, which I had previously ignored, and these gave me an altered conceptual framework of 'those patterns of thinking, feeling, believing, and behavior that animate our lives' (Green 2008, p.98). This new broader framework became the basis for re-evaluating aspects of my sense of self (Bryan 2016, p.19). Although intellect was still of paramount importance to me, I began to appreciate emotional and spiritual aspects of my self. These became increasingly important, as I tried to handle the very negative impact of the dementia diagnosis.

In contrast to the experience of conversion, in which I had discovered positive aspects of a sense of self within a community, diagnosis was a negative and extremely isolating event. My cognition – my intellect – was threatened by diagnosis, and the idea of a loss of self with dementia led to an overwhelming fear of future non-being. This was an existential fear, 'the anxiety of not being able to preserve one's own being' (Tillich 1969, p.47). How could I remain Christine, if my brain was disappearing and I was slowly losing my sharp intellect? My sense of self was so bound up with my ability to think and reason, that I spiralled downhill with despair, unable to rise above negative thinking about my future.

In one of my first talks after diagnosis, I described 'the toxic power of the "pointing bone" of diagnosis… [resulting in] extreme fear of further loss, and dread [of] what the future holds' (Bryden 2015b, p.20). I spoke of how I felt cast out into what felt like the valley of the shadow of death (p.19). Diagnosis was my absolute lowest point, yet eventually I was able to find some comfort in my newfound faith community. I was so very thankful to have discovered a new sense of an emotional and spiritual self within this community. I began to regard cognitive ability as perhaps being less important than an ability to relate to others and to what was giving me a new sense of meaning. However, I was still on occasion overwhelmed by fear, as the story of loss of self seemed to permeate all discussion of dementia, and oppress those of us struggling to live as best we could with this condition.

Who would I be when I died with dementia? Even my understanding of my newfound faith was tinged with doubts and fears. Although I was reassured that God's move towards humanity lies at the heart of the Christian faith, my understanding was caught between my conversion *experience*, and my search for *knowledge*. I felt that I needed more knowledge, and was focused at that time on knowing about God, rather than knowing God. I was trying to explore faith through the lens of knowledge and of intellect.

My fears after diagnosis were exacerbated by the very common dualist view of what I thought it meant to be a self: a person with a mortal brain/body and an immortal spirit. This is a view that has persisted from the times of the Greek philosophers, and indeed even impacted on the thinking of early Christian thinkers. Believing this view, I thought I was made up of a brain/body and an immortal soul/spirit, and this dualist view added to my fears of my brain being the key to my self. As my brain disappeared gradually over time, resulting in dementia, I might become a mindless shell and an immortal spirit. What would that mean? How could I exist in the world around me, just as a spirit without a brain or mind? I now realise that I had misunderstood what the word *mind* meant, believing that it was reliant on having an intact brain. I had a very limited understanding of a more holistic view of self, which was affecting my perception of my future, and which had a particularly negative impact on my reaction to a diagnosis of dementia.

4

Challenging Loss of Self in Dementia

Hannah had now been living with dementia for a few years. She was going regularly for testing, in a windowless room with a clinician who showed absolutely no emotion. She could not tell if she had guessed the right answer or not. The blank walls gave her no clues as to ideas for objects starting with 'P' or for remembering a shopping list of bizarre objects all listed together. Each year there was always some surprise, as she had forgotten some aspect of the test. But as to living with dementia itself, maybe she was getting used to it? Hannah's main concern was her role as the mainstay of the home. Would she be able to remember all the rituals of the Shabat? She was sure that her daughter, Rachel, would help her, but when would her mind disappear? When would her beloved daughter and husband, David, have to face up to her 'departure'? Would she really disintegrate as a human being, and be unable to know Rachel or David? What a terrible future awaited her when that happened! It seemed as if her doctors could not tell her how long she had until those awful things might happen to her – would it be months or years? But David's love shone out of his eyes and she knew that he would stay alongside her in this journey. At the moment she was enjoying book club and knitting, as well as tennis group, and all her friends still seemed to accept her for who she was. They included her in their activities, even if she had forgotten events coming up and needed to be reminded of them. She loved to look at all the photos of her family on the mantelpiece, and see how big all the dear grandchildren were getting. Would she live to see them grow to be young men and women, married with their own children?

In my previous books, I have described the trauma of my diagnosis with dementia, resulting from my view at the time that brain equals mind equals self: therefore a gradual loss of my brain would mean loss of self. This fear was very much underpinned by my focus on the importance of my intellect as the source of my identity. For example, I wrote, 'Having a disease which takes away your mind' (Bryden 2012, p.97) and 'As I travel towards the dissolution of my self' (Bryden and MacKinlay 2002, p.74). These words clearly demonstrate how I believed the all-pervasive idea in society that I would lose my self to dementia.

Can you imagine what it must feel like to be told you have dementia, while being surrounded by assumptions of loss of self, and even to believe them yourself? Even those organisations supposed to help us once had terrible views; dementia was described as a condition where 'the mind is absent and the body an empty shell' (Alzheimer's Disease International 2000, p.1). This bleak picture of loss is also often mentioned by care-partners, who speak of facing the so-called 'departure of a loved one' (Kevern 2010, p.238). Would my family be facing my 'departure' and, if so, where would I be going? Would I really be leaving an empty shell behind?

All these views about loss of self that surround us mean that we become 'imprisoned in a web of negative stereotypes' (Sabat *et al.* 2011, p.286), where assumptions are made about our lack of capability, and that we will eventually become a terrible burden for our care-partners. Dementia is accompanied by stigma, and everyone becomes awkward around us because they fear that we might show embarrassing behaviours. Society values competence, intelligence and autonomy, and devalues those of us who might be unable to demonstrate these attributes. Therefore, the belief that we are losing these abilities can result in our isolation, so that 'we live within a complex web of social encounters that are tainted with stigma' (Bryden 2015b, p.111). If people are experiencing problems with cognition, they even defer seeking a diagnosis, because of their fear of a loss of self with dementia. Others, when diagnosed, *even consider euthanasia*, as a way of avoiding what they think will be an inescapable loss of self. This is why is it so important to challenge these views of loss of self in dementia, which lead to stigma, isolation and fears of the future, to give people being diagnosed (and their families) hope for the present and the future.

Doctors think in terms of the biomedical picture of there being cognitive decline, as measured by neuropsychological tests and brain scans. These diagnostic tests are carried out in a sterile environment, where there is no relationship with the clinician. However, we all function best as communal beings: 'Human beings do not exist in a vacuum, in isolation, yet sometimes, the way that dementia is defined in the biomedical paradigm, this would seem to be the case' (MacKinlay 2016, p.33). How can my sense of self be measured, if my relationships are ignored? Human beings cannot be tested in environments devoid of relationships: none of us lives in isolation from the rest of humanity (Allen and Coleman 2006, p.213).

I have great communicative difficulties in neuropsychological testing, where I struggle to find the words I need and am not helped by the clinician looking down at her notes, rather than at me. I cannot use hand gestures or facial expressions to convey my thoughts, and must rely on my increasingly problematic word finding. My communication is being 'interpreted as being "dispositional," or due to [my] way of being, rather than "situational," or due to the circumstances' of the clinical environment (Sabat and Lee 2011, p.316). My cognition is being measured in a situation of stress and anxiety, instead of in a rich social context, so is not representative of my normal abilities. Indeed if *anyone* were to be tested in such a clinical environment, I suggest they might experience some unexpected difficulties! Therefore 'people with dementia cannot and should not be positioned as incapable of acting as social beings on the basis of their cognitive test scores' (Sabat and Lee 2011, p.324). Instead, we should be observed in situations similar to everyday life, which is 'lived in rich social, interpersonal context that go far beyond the quality of the interpersonal relationship between a test-giver and test-taker' (Sabat and Gladstone 2010, p.73).

The result of testing is that we become described by a set of standard cognitive defects, where the 'clinical approach assumes that our brains, our life histories and our individual life experiences are all the same' (Bryden 2015b, p.204). However, each one of us is a unique person, and the brain is a key part of what makes us very special. How can damage to the brain be thought of in the same way as damage to a bone, for example? The brain is individually 'wired up' over a lifetime to make us who we are; it is adaptable and extremely complex. But when we have dementia, all this is cast aside and we are no longer respected as unique people; everything about us is due to neurological loss. No consideration is given to how we might be able to overcome this loss of brain matter, such as by encouraging *neuroplasticity*, which is discussed in Norman Doidge's book *The Brain That Changes Itself* (2007). This is the ability of the brain to compensate for damage, taking up functions in other less damaged parts, through rehabilitative exercises after such events as stroke and traumatic brain injury.

Doctors focus only on what we can no longer do, not on what we still can do or could be encouraged to do, and highlight only our deficiencies. This has been described as 'defectology' (Swinton 2012, pp.41–43), where we 'have lost not only our identity, but also our diversity. Everything that once made us a unique…individual with value to society, has been lost' (Bryden 2015b, p.274). In this regard, theologian John Swinton refers to the novel *Scar Tissue*, in which a philosopher professor loves his mother for *who she is*, despite her dementia, in contrast with his neurologist brother who only sees *what is being lost*. This shows 'a disjunction and a tension between medical accounts of dementia and the lived experiences of dementia' (Swinton 2012, p.33).

Shortly after diagnosis, I was shocked to read theologian David Keck's words that a loss of memory might lead to the 'apparent disintegration of a human being' (1996, p.15), dementia being 'Destruction Incarnate' (p.21), and 'when there is no self, there can be little self-realization' (p.38). I sought a counter-story to challenge Keck's view of dementia. How could I possibly be disintegrating as a human being, solely due to the slow deterioration of my brain? I wrote:

We are each a kaleidoscope of personality, which makes up every facet of who we are. But often we are limited in our range of expression of this multi-faceted person, because of our busy-ness, the demands and constraints, the expectations of our lives… as this disease unwraps me, opens up the treasures of what lies within my multi-fold personality, I can feel safe as each layer is gently opened out… In each of these aspects of my life, the centre of my being will always be there, expressing itself in these many forms of me. This unique essence of 'me' is at my core, and this is what will remain with me to the end. I will be perhaps even more truly 'me' than I have ever been. (Bryden 2012, pp.62, 64)

I knew that I had become slower, less vibrant and more disconnected in my thought processes, and yet I still felt there was more to me. I was less cognitive, but retained an emotional and spiritual sense of self, so I began to see my dementia as a stripping away of masks: of my cognitive work self, then an increasingly jumbled emotional self, towards my 'true' self (Bryden 2005, p.159).

5

'I Who Know That I Exist Inquire Into What I Am'

Gerald had been living with dementia for some years now, and still felt like himself. He simply could not understand why he had been so worried about the so-called loss of self that he thought would happen after he had been diagnosed. It still had not happened! He would look down at his body and see his gradually ageing legs, arms and torso. They might be getting a bit wrinklier over time, but that was quite normal. His partner Fred was still there to reassure him; they had been a couple for so long now and their loving relationship was a key part of who Gerald felt he was. Fred and Gerald still enjoyed the things they always had done – BBQs on the beach, as well as visits to art galleries to contemplate the beauty of the various works. Fred knew how much art meant to Gerald, and how he could spend ages sitting in front of a painting, contemplating it and gaining a deep sense of meaning. Dementia had not impacted on any of this enjoyment at all. Gerald was quite aware of what was not himself in the world around him, so felt sure he could distinguish self from non-self. There was no way he thought he was a chair, for example! How ridiculous to think he would lose his sense of self and think he was a piece of furniture, rather than Fred's partner for life! He was also able to relate to their circle of friends; mind you, they were doing a lot more of the 'relating' nowadays, as he was forgetting all of their names, as well as what had happened in their lives. Often Fred would quietly prompt him so that he could make some sensible comment or ask a sympathetic question. But Gerald still knew that their friends were people with kind faces; it was just their labels he had lost, and their stories. He could not attach a label or a story to a face – it was all a bit of a jumble. But nothing had changed in the way Gerald looked and smiled at people, and he hoped they would reciprocate. Gerald really struggled to recall a lot of things in his life; what he had done last week, let alone last year or a few years ago, and he would be quite lost without Fred. When he looked at photo albums, he needed Fred's help to work out who was who. When he tried to talk to people, it was so hard to tell them his story, but he could talk in the present moment about what he found interesting and meaningful.

The philosopher René Descartes writes, 'I am conscious that I exist, and I who know that I exist inquire into what I am' (1637/1912, p.88). This quote is a good description of what I am writing about in this book, as I know I exist and I am enquiring into what or who I am. However, the usual view is that, because of my dementia, I should be unable to do this, due to my decreasing cognitive abilities.

Descartes' view was that the body is separate from the mind – known as Cartesian dualism – and he made the well-known statement 'I think therefore I am.' This challenges those of us with dementia, whose thoughts are becoming more muddled. However, Descartes' view contrasts with modern Christian views of a holistic view of being, in which we are 'psychophysical unities' (Murphy 2006, p.22). Nowadays, scientists also often describe the brain in terms of a similar dualism, when they make claims about what the brain can do or perceive. This scientific dualism is criticised by Sabat (2010), who points out that we are not a body *and* a mind, but a whole living human being, with bodily, spiritual and psychological capacity.

It is important to combat dualism in order to cast aside the assumption that, as my brain deteriorates, so does my sense of self. It is in and through my body (including my brain) that I express my inward/outward life. My brain is part of, not separate from my body: it never was separate, and grew alongside my body, so cannot be taken out and placed in a laboratory to see if it senses or feels anything. How could it possibly do so, without all the sensory organs that I have in the rest of my body?

Many people argue that a loss of sense of self occurs at some time during the lived experience of dementia, and might ask how I could know what might happen much later on in my journey with dementia. But I have been with people in the later and last stages of dementia, as well as with many others who are living with dementia as best they can, and have developed a very different view: as embodied relational selves, we can continue to find meaningful narratives in the present moment. If people with dementia are assumed to experience a loss of self, we are at risk of less than optimal care, as we are then thought of as being little more than empty shells. I want to turn around these views, so that people with dementia are respected as having a continuing sense of self throughout dementia. *It is a whole person who is being related to and cared for, not some physical presence from which the self has departed.*

I am a heart and body, as much as I am a brain, able to relate to others and to the world. My sense of self cannot be measured by examining neurological defects, as I also have thoughts, images or fleeting pictures in my mind even if I can't describe them, and feelings, although I am losing the ability to express these clearly. Importantly, I know who I am, and have the ability to distinguish self from non-self. My inability to recall or express information has no impact on this sense of self; yet being able to do this is important in what ethicist Stephen Post refers to as our 'hypercognitive culture' (1995, p.5). In this description of modern society, our worth is measured by what we know, do and say, and by what we achieve in regard to expectations of rationalism and productivity. These expectations of being an autonomous and rational individual challenge those of us whose cognition is failing.

My cognitive abilities might be decreasing, yet I continue to have a sense of embodiment, in relationships with others and with what gives me a sense of meaning. I am the self, knower, subject and agent for my thoughts, which occur in relationships with others around me. There has been no disruption at any time since diagnosis to my subjective sense of being Christine. I have not become, nor do I feel as if I am becoming, someone else because of dementia, and I have a stable sense of self that has continued from before my diagnosis, right through to now. Post is critical of any suggestion that there is a lack of stability of self before and after diagnosis as any attempt to split the self into 'then' and 'now' is, in his view, 'nonsense'. I am still the same self, and will remain so throughout my lived experience of dementia, 'despite behaviour and communication having changed' (Allen and Coleman 2006, p.206). Why should problems with my recall, sense of time or language diminish my sense of self? I continue to be 'me' and to see the world through 'my' eyes, in the present moment. From this insider's viewpoint, I know that I am the same self who existed a while ago: even if I cannot remember the facts or feelings of what I did or felt at that time, this does not mean that I have lost my sense of who I am.

In today's Western society, having a *thinking self* is usually associated with having an intact brain, giving rise to the view that the increasing brain damage that leads to dementia will indeed mean a loss of self. A thinking self is described by philosopher Locke as the ability to keep track of the self at different times and places (1975), giving a continuing sense of personal identity over time. Locke assumes that memory is the fundamental aspect of this identity, so that we only remain the same person over time if we have a chain of memories to link us back. This is of concern, as I am indeed losing the ability to keep track of myself at different times and places, because I cannot recall what happened last week or last month, let alone last year, without help. Therefore I accept that I do have a loss of a 'thinking self' (Holton 2016, p.256), which is often of central concern for those of us with dementia. Will our chain of memories become broken and, if we have no help with recall, who will we become? But I am arguing for *a self that is far more than simply the ability to keep track*, but is able to have a sense of embodiment, be in relationships and find meaning.

I lack the ability to recall all the moments to trace events over time, but I can do this with help to access the filing cabinet of my memories, which are increasingly difficult to recover without aid. Recall is what is difficult, not the underlying memories themselves, which remain in a jumbled, mixed-up pile, rather than filed in some sort of order. However, there is so much more to me than an accurate recall of a chain of events and keeping track of my self at different times and places. A focus on the so-called thinking self can be taken to an extreme to highlight its absurdity: while we are asleep, we are unable to keep track of ourselves, but when we wake up we still have a sense of self (Holton 2016, p.258). I wake up each day and still feel like Christine, even if I do not know what day it is or what happened yesterday! I still continue as 'me' in the present moment, despite being unable to trace my sense of self accurately over time, without help.

Perspectives on loss of self in dementia have come from outside observers, who can only imagine whether this actually occurs; *they cannot know.* The voices of people with dementia are more recently becoming heard, telling their story. Who am I, as I struggle with recall over time: who will I become as my brain deteriorates further? One day, will I cease to be me? From my insider's viewpoint, I know that I am an 'I', and this 'I' is inquiring into who 'I' am. What is the self and is it solely due to the brain? How can the brain give a subjective awareness of the world? To what extent has science, philosophy, psychology or theology advanced our understanding? Can I counter the modern view of the neurological primacy of the brain as the seat of the self?

6

Embodied Self

Chabi was scared of the world around her, as it was all becoming so strange. But when she looked down she could still see the familiar body that she had lived in all these years, even though it was ageing. As she moved into the living room, she wondered who this old man was – how could he possibly be her husband, Abhay, like he often said he was? Her husband was a younger, more handsome man, although this older man was friendly and very helpful, looking at her with love in his eyes. There were other people around the table, and this man who said he was her husband told her all their names, saying they were her children. Surely not – they were far too old! But Abhay was wonderful, helping her to cope, even with cooking and getting things ready, so that no one really noticed what a struggle these sorts of gatherings were becoming. Chabi felt so much better when they all left, when she and this very kind man could relax. The funny thing was she had no doubt that she was still Chabi, but the big mirror in their wardrobe gave her a huge shock one day. She screamed in fear at the strange person walking towards her – who was this intruder? No matter what Abhay said, it didn't make it any better, so he covered up the big wardrobe mirror with an old sari. Chabi could now go into their wardrobe with no problems at all, and really couldn't understand what the fuss had been about. She just wondered why Abhay was using her old sari like that.

My sense of being an embodied self includes living with dementia, as this is who I am, as well as who I will be until I die. I have a sense of being embodied as an 'I' with first-person feelings about the world around me, distinguishing self from non-self. The view of outsiders as to whether I am still 'me' presumes that I have forgotten who 'I' am, and that with a loss of language and of recall, a sense of self is lost. For example, Swinton writes, 'Am "I" still "me" when "I" have forgotten who "I" am?' (2012, p.91). However, my sense of self continues, despite me being unable to keep track of memories because of 'the erosion of the temporal glue' (Post 2006, p.225). This is a great phrase to describe the sieve in my brain, which makes it increasingly difficult to recall things. But even if my recollection of taking my tablets a few moments ago has gone, or I cannot find the word for tablets, I still exist as 'me' in the present moment. My lack of recall has not affected my sense of being embodied in the moment – and, indeed, why should it? I might forget writing this bit of the book tomorrow, but why should this mean a loss of 'me'?

My sense of being an embodied self continues within dementia: I see the world through my own eyes, and it is 'that part of me when I am with myself' (Reinders 2008, p.21). My sense of being Christine remains intact in dementia, despite my disrupted sense of time and my linguistic, thought ordering and recall dysfunctions. Although I am losing capacities to express my sense of self, due to my language becoming more muddled and confused, I still have unique personal characteristics, which are not lost because of failing cognition. This uniqueness is not impacted by my need for an increasing amount of help to recall what happened last week, last month or last year, or to recall what I am planning today, next week or next month. I feel disconnected in time, without the anchor of accurate recall, and so cannot travel back and forth in time in my 'mind's eye' to develop a better picture of my comings and goings. I feel as if I have lost my ability to travel in time, so that sometimes I feel as if I could benefit from a 'time machine' to give me a glimpse of a time that has passed or one that is being anticipated! My sense of being increasingly adrift on a timeline means that I am losing a reliable connection with my past, and to the future; yet I am still the Christine who, even without language, has the *feelings* of 'What is happening to me?'

I might be 'all at sea' in terms of recall, but I will always continue as an embodied self who can be addressed as 'you' and who asks the question: 'Who am I?' My experience of being an embodied self is very similar to the *Self 1* described by Sabat: my self of personal identity, who thinks of her experiences and beliefs in the first person (Sabat 2001, pp.17–18). This social constructionist definition includes the *Self 1* of my personal identity, which is experienced as my point of view and expressed through the use of personal pronouns. It also includes the *Self 2* of my unique mental and physical attributes, such as being a former scientist and policy advisor, and having a diagnosis of dementia. I am aware of changes to my *Self 2*, due to the decline I am experiencing with dementia, so I feel despair at 'who I am not, but might otherwise be' (Sabat 2001, p.117).

Importantly, my sense of embodiment also includes the *Self 3* of personality and character, which is how others see me in social interactions. These outsiders' perceptions impact on my experiences profoundly, as I am often surrounded by negative views of dementia. Therefore my constant struggle is not only to battle with my own neurological deficits, but also with the stigma of dementia: the story of loss of self, and the negativity around me in society. It is very important that our personalities, characters and how others see us are not placed at risk, as this can result in negative positioning of people with dementia in social encounters (Swinton 2012, p.89), in which we are stripped of all other descriptors of our lives. We are far more than a person with dementia, and have rich personalities and characters worthy of being respected. I have written, 'Maintain our dignity and avoid depersonalizing us' (Bryden 2015b, p.224).

I sense that I continue to exist, moment to moment, relative to my surroundings, and can express this by saying 'I', 'me' and 'my' to locate myself in my psychosocial world. Recognising my continuing sense of being an embodied self within dementia is important for those on the outside, so that they can regard me as having a valid *subjective* perspective, which is my insider's view, giving new insights into the lived experience of dementia. As Post writes,

'What is morally relevant is the experience of subjectivity, of myself as a subject in the sense of being conscious of self as self' (2006, p.230). My sense of being an embodied self, who is sitting here writing this part of my book, is the same embodied self that sat here a moment ago, even if I cannot recall that moment. Many people might find it hard to believe that I could write like this, and yet not recall that I sat down to write a day or so ago. But *this is my reality*, this sense of being a continuing embodied self, who I am, then and now, and my damaged brain has not diminished this sense of being present.

Scientific views of embodiment

What can science tell us about the self? What we know from science is about the brain, not the self, and even then it is impossible to study the human brain in isolation from the body in the laboratory. As Christian physicist John Polkinghorne observes: 'there is an ugly big ditch yawning between scientific accounts of the firings of neural networks…and the simplest mental experience of perceiving a patch of pink' (1996, p.53). Scientists themselves are using their own brains to study the phenomenon of self. Surely it is problematic to use the subject of the study for the investigations and conclusions? How can a brain study itself and identify facts and evidence for what it means, for example, to perceive a patch of pink? How do I know that you perceive this patch in the same way?

I am not a brain in a laboratory, but a whole person situated in my body, of which the brain is but one part.

My brain and my body developed together, and my brain cannot be separated from my body. The nerves to and from the brain reach all the body's sensory organs, giving the brain information about the environment, as well as delivering information to the body. If you cut these nerves to put the brain in a laboratory, there is nothing to see, hear, taste or touch. Sabat critiques the attribution of aspects of psychological experience to parts of the brain, where researchers write that the brain perceives this or that. He emphasises that the brain is a part of the body and cannot operate alone, and notes how this is 'creating a new form of Cartesian dualism' (Sabat 2010, p.168).

The deterioration of the brain that results in dementia does not mean a loss of self, as the brain is not the self, nor can it interpret or do anything. My brain and my body act in concert: they both arrived in this world together and then I began to perceive what was around me. I have developed awareness about what is exterior to my body, and what is part of it; in that sense, my thoughts and bodily perceptions are included in my sense of embodied self. The brain cannot give me this sense of self, as it is only one part of who I am as a whole unique person of intrinsic value, or 'a unity that is compiled of different facets', such as my embodied existence and my experience of the world around me (Sabat 2010, p.174).

In order to explore my sense of embodiment, the ideas of the neurobiologist Antonio Damasio are helpful. His work is well informed by brain research, and he proposes that created within deep brain structures is a *proto-self* (Damasio 2010, pp.20–21), which gives me my feelings of existence prior to my consciousness arising. Damasio suggests that this proto-self provides an integrated collection of neural patterns within and about my body (p.190), interpreting the world, interacting with my brain and having primordial feelings. Next to arise is the *core self* that modifies this proto-self to provide a series of images and is able to distinguish self from non-self, and 'constitutes a material "me"' (pp.20–23). This is the embodied self that I refer to, which can distinguish self from non-self. I am still able to see the world through my own eyes, knowing I am Christine, and having feelings about what is happening to me as I live with dementia.

My view is that, throughout the process of brain deterioration that results in dementia, the deep brain structures referred to by Damasio as producing a sense of existence are resistant. The persistence of these deep structures, despite ongoing brain damage, means that I can have a continuing sense of being an embodied self, with feelings of existence, separate from my surroundings. Nevertheless, Damasio refers to people in the late stages of dementia as being 'shells of the human beings they once were' (2010, p.233). This is an outsider's view of people with dementia, and appears to contradict his idea of a self that emerges from deep brain structures and that should remain, despite the brain damage resulting in dementia. How can I become a shell, if my proto or core self remains deep within my brain stem? In contrast, I suggest that both the proto-self and core self remain throughout dementia, dependent on the persistence of the brain stem, and give rise to a continuing sense of being an embodied self.

I might have reduced recall of past events and difficulties with language, but I still have consciousness, awareness of self and non-self, as well as feelings, imagery and a sense of embodiment.

Other neuroscientists (Matyushkin 2008) also hypothesise a neurophysiological basis of self, and their views agree with the available data and the ideas of Damasio. In these studies, the existence of a lower self, based on a subcortical neuronal network, is confirmed by some experimental electrical stimulation studies and correlates with Damasio's proposed core self. My view is that the core self persists despite ongoing brain damage to give a continuing sense of self.

Scientific views of recall dysfunction

The term memory loss is often used in dementia but, as I have written earlier, this is more correctly referred to as recall dysfunction, as my memories remain, but I need additional prompts to recall them. A problem with recall is an important feature of dementia, yet the neurological architecture for this difficulty is not well understood. We appear to perceive, learn and manipulate information in an interaction of neuronal pathways to interpret, record and perceive events, which is based on complex patterns for storage and mechanisms of access in a network of maps and images (Damasio 2010, p.135). Given this complexity, at least some of these neuronal pathways might persist in dementia, so as to account for the retention of *procedural* (knowhow), as well as aspects of *semantic* (conceptual) memory. This might explain the so-called 'lucid episodes' observed by care-partners (Aquilina and Hughes 2006, p.145). Importantly, our memories lie deep within, able to be accessed when we are helped to recall them.

What is feared most in dementia is a loss of *episodic* memory, or an ability to recall past events without help, as the outsider's perception is that this means loss of self. However, this assumes that my sense of being an embodied self is dependent on recalling what I did, rather than on *knowing who I am*. Why should the ability to retain memories be regarded as so critical to having a sense of self? Why should a lack of accurate and reliable recall of past events mean that I am losing myself? Surely, I still retain a sense of who I am, and have a sense of the true meaning of what it means to be Christine? Indeed, I suggest a robot could be programmed to recall accurately the entire record of its 'life', yet it cannot be regarded to know what it is, or to have a sense of meaning. I wonder why a lack of a remembered timeline is so important to outsiders, who then regard me as having 'lost my self'?

My experience is that, within my neurological architecture, prompts can provide access to neuronal pathways. An experimental verification for the persistence of recall for past events, potentially due to the retention of deep brain structures and neural pathways, is the finding of Sabat that people with dementia could be prompted to retrieve some recall of past events (2001, p.45). I use a variety of prompts to assist in recall, which 'is as if the printer ink is running low and it sometimes works and sometimes doesn't… It is such a hit and miss approach to a life gone by' (Bryden 2005, p.106). For example, I use a personal calendar application on my phone, tablet and computer, so as to remain oriented to the current day, past events, as well as future plans. If someone rings to ask how yesterday was, I can look it up in the calendar and be engaged in the conversation. If instead they ask if I am looking forward to next week, once again I can participate by checking my calendar: 'if something is not written in the diary it has not happened or will not happen. Ask me how my day was and I'll have to look at the diary and find out' (Bryden 2015b, p.130).

By seeing what is written, I am given a chance to recognise an event and to be able to retrieve it. This appears to be *recognition* memory, reliant on an external prompt, rather than episodic memory that accurately recalls the flow of events over time. However, on many occasions, I see only words on the calendar and cannot actually form a memory or a picture in my mind. It seems as if my past and future have become devoid of events, and I have a mental blank; as if a black curtain has fallen down behind and before me, so that although I can retrieve some factual events from my calendar, these are just words, not images in my mind. *Nonetheless, I still have a sense of self.*

Philosophical views of embodiment

Among modern philosophical accounts of the embodied self are arguments for causal reductionism, in which I am 'nothing but' my neurones. This reductionism gives rise to the conclusion that dementia due to brain damage leads to a loss of self, which has been a dominant position, particularly among atheistic scientists. The Christian philosopher Nancey Murphy (1998) offers an alternative, which takes into account contemporary scientific views, such as those of Damasio. She has developed the concept of nonreductive physicalism, which suggests that I am far more than 'nothing but' my neurones, and have a sense of self. Nonreductive physicalism gives an explanation for my capacity for emotion, morality and spirituality, without recourse to body–spirit dualism, and goes beyond the idea of 'bottom-up' causation of my actions (or reductionism), to include downward causation, so I cannot be reduced to brain damage alone. My higher level capacities are dependent on lower level processes, yet also causative in their own right, emerging from complex interactions of the entire brain. Presumably these lower level processes occur within deep brain structures, resistant to the brain damage resulting in dementia, which is similar to my conclusion from Damasio's approach to the core self arising in these structures.

Complex patterns of interaction with the environment have effects on the developing brain in 'a dynamic interplay between neurobiology and environment' (Murphy 2006, p.101), which includes evaluating cognitive processes in a process that Murphy calls 'self-transcendence' (p.89). Murphy's concept of nonreductive physicalism is consistent with Damasio's (2010) idea of a dynamic relationship between my deeply embedded proto-self and the environment, resulting in a core self. These concepts can reassure me by accounting for a continuing sense of embodied self in dementia.

However, Murphy (2006, p.95) discusses the ability to distinguish self from non-self, and quotes from analytical philosopher Patricia Churchland (2002, p.309) that such capacities for self-representation emerge in children and *decline in people with dementia*. Concurring with Churchland's view appears to counter Murphy's own arguments of the complexity of the entire brain, and that I am more than my neurones (Murphy 2006, p.151). I disagree with the idea that there is a decline in this ability to distinguish self from non-self in people with dementia. If I am more than my neurones, as Murphy proposes, how can I lose my concept of self on the basis of a loss of some of these brain cells? Churchland herself refers to Damasio's proto-self as the non-conscious platform for higher levels of self-representation (2002, p.310), which accords with Murphy's reasoning that a higher level capacity is dependent on lower level processes.

The three thinkers, Damasio, Murphy and Churchland, have not explored my view concerning the possible persistence of deep brain structures throughout dementia for giving a continuing sense of self. In addition, there needs to be further consideration of the neuroplasticity of the brain in the face of assaults to its structure (Doidge 2007). Certainly, I have experienced a degree of such neuroplasticity occurring since my diagnosis, as a result of continuing to challenge my brain, such as by writing this book. My conclusion is that dementia should not take away my sense of embodiment, as I am far more than my decreasing neurones; I can rely on my life experiences, as well as deep brain structures, for a continuing sense of embodied self, even through the ongoing loss of neurones and neural pathways.

Retention of embodied virtues

Pauline had a delightful room on the first floor of a lovely care home, which was a former stately house with beautiful grounds. Downstairs was the dining room and also a sitting room, overlooking the lawns. The dining tables were laid for meals with damask tablecloths and silverware, and there was sherry on the sideboard before dinner. Pauline couldn't recall how long she had been there, nor why she had moved there, but perhaps it was because when she had been at home she had been finding it hard to cope? Remembering things had become very difficult, such as taking tablets, or making breakfast or dinner, let alone getting up and down those stairs. Even the stairlift was becoming harder to work out how to use! It had become far too overwhelming. Her wonderful daughter, Janet, had arranged for her to go into this home, which was in the village where she lived, so she popped in most days. Pauline loved to help the others who were there in the home, who needed to get up from or down to the table or find the lift. This gave her a deep sense of purpose and meaning. She had made quite a few friends here now, and had found a new lease of life in discovering just how much she could do for others. The staff also appreciated everything Pauline did, especially on outings such as the one where she had been the one to choose the rescue cat for the home. Each evening she would put on her delicate pearl necklace, which made her feel very special. It was from her dear husband, Clive, so in a way he was there with her every day. She would often look at his photo by her bedside – what a handsome man he had been! Pauline would go down in the lift for dinner, where they all gathered for a glass of sherry and looked at the lovely view. This was certainly the best place to be, if you couldn't be at home! In fact, in some ways it was better, because she had been very lonely and isolated at home, and here she had found purpose in helping others and making friends!

Virtues are an important feature of the continuing embodied self, as described by Sabat for *Self 2* (2001, pp.17–18). We each have deeply ingrained habits and ways of interacting with others. For example, the retention of virtues has been observed amongst residents of a care facility, who demonstrated mutual care, compassion and concern (McFadden, Ingram and Baldauf 2000, p.80). Similarly, Sabat finds the persistence of virtues in his conversations with people with dementia (2001, pp.307–308), such as Dr B., who expressed concerns over Sabat's wellbeing (p.56). These observations are also supported by an abstract philosophical thought experiment described by Murphy, which shows the importance to a person of a sense of self over time that is not only a continuing mix of embodiment, but also, importantly, a persistence of virtues (Murphy 2006, p.137).

The philosopher Alasdair MacIntyre discusses virtues, highlighting giving and receiving in a network of relationships as a virtue of interdependence (1999, p.108). He proposes that providing care demonstrates the virtue of independent rational agency, and receiving care the virtue of acknowledged dependence (p.85). Indeed, we all have a mix of both virtues in our relationships. MacIntyre's statement that 'I can be said truly to know who and what I am, only because there are others who can be said to truly know who and what I am' succinctly suggests the importance of relationships (p.95). Relationships are critical to us all, particularly for people with dementia, a point which I consider in the following chapter.

7

Relational self

Jai had been living with dementia for a few years now, and was struggling more with words, recall and the way time seemed to flit to and fro. But his wife, Hari, was wonderful, and would always be there, helping him in everything, including when he tried to speak or recall things. Very few people noticed his problems because of the way Hari was able to help him, remembering events, quietly prompting him about their friends' lives, as well as with getting dressed, when even his turban was becoming more of a problem. Hari's cooking was delicious and even seemed to rival the wonderful scents that welcomed him in the Gurdwara! Hari knew that Jai's friendships were very important to him, and she helped him with quiet prompts if he had forgotten who someone was or what was happening in their lives. And amongst the congregational gathering, Jai felt welcomed, accepted and as if his problems had somehow disappeared. He wasn't trying to relate to others on the basis of knowledge, but was being welcomed as an equal. He could still smile, nod and acknowledge others in these relationships.

Dementia is a complex interaction between neurological impairment and social interaction, which is as 'much a relational disability as it is a physical or neurological one' (Swinton 2011, p.177). The importance of relationships to us all is expressed very well by Post, who writes 'I feel and relate, and therefore, I am' (2006, p.233), which is in stark contrast to Descartes's dictum 'I think, therefore I am' (1637/1912, p.168). A focus on thinking, rather than relating, can exclude people with dementia, but by exploring my embodied *relational* self, the difficulties due to cognitive impairment can be overcome.

My relational self is a sense of being an embodied self in relationships with others, so that I am aware of my body, and can see others around me who are connecting with me, often without words. They can compensate for my problems with language and recall, as well as support me so that I can still feel accepted and welcomed. Indeed, we are all embodied selves who relate to one another as an 'I' and recognise an 'I', which does not need cognitive ability such as language. When I meet a Japanese friend, we become 'we' as two selves, despite having no common language. We relate to each other, and between us is a connection without words. I have found that I can relate to Japanese friends through eye contact and touch. One example of such a deep connection occurred when we were visiting a day care centre in Matsue, Japan. I was crouching down in front of a lady in her mid-90s, who was seated on one of a line of chairs ready to meet me. This lady had long ago lost her ability to speak, and looked gloomily down at her lap. I touched her hands, looked into her eyes, and spoke in

English for a while, trying to communicate with her. At last I felt the pressure of her gnarled old fingers, as she grasped my hand tightly and looked back into my eyes. This was the spark of a relationship, across culture and across language, without the need for words to communicate meaning. How can we ever say that relationships rely on cognition?

I do not have the same cognitive capacity as I once had, yet still have a sense of embodiment as an 'I' who is present, relating to others in the world. My 'I' connects 'me' over time, including a material, social and spiritual 'me', to create a sense of continuity. My social 'me' is formed in relationships with others; my spiritual 'me' is developed in connection with what gives me a sense of meaning, so that I have developed a sense of being a storied spiritual being (Poll and Smith 2003, p.130). This is the same across the faiths, and indeed for people of no faith. Some of us gain a sense of meaning from a particular religion, which connects us with rituals and beliefs that can lift our spirit, and give us a feeling of becoming connected with the divine. Others amongst us gain a sense of meaning from nature or art, so that we feel deeply touched by contemplating a work of art, such as music, painting or ballet, or from activities such as walking, golf or tennis that take us out into the beauty of nature. Young children can also give a sense of meaning, in their unconditional acceptance and happy chatter around their elderly relatives.

For me, my Christian faith gives me a sense of meaning, and I do not feel any less me because of my steady decline due to dementia. There have been, and continue to be, important learnings into this journey of increasing impairment. However, although my ability to perform spiritual practices, and to remember and describe them to others, is being impacted, my 'inherent holiness is not affected by neurological decline' (Swinton 2012, p.174). Outsiders can gain a mistaken impression that I am no longer able to appreciate what gives me a sense of meaning, because I am less able to describe my experiences. However, from my insider's viewpoint, I know that I do not need fully functioning neuronal pathways to have a sense of being an embodied spiritual me. I agree with theologian Ray Anderson who wrote that the 'existence of brain cells is a necessary but insufficient condition for the expression of...spiritual being' (1998, p.188). We can have a spiritual self-identity, despite a deteriorating brain.

Relating to what gives us a sense of meaning

Ghazala looked carefully into the mirror as she dressed for prayers this Friday. Today she needed more help from her daughter, Tahera, as this was all getting much harder for her. When she had first been diagnosed with dementia, she had thought it would just mean a bit of memory loss, but now she was realising all sorts of things were becoming more difficult. The latest problems she was experiencing were in fixing her hijab correctly, so Ghazala was very glad that Tahera still lived at home, as she was able to help her, as well as take her to prayer in the women's chamber of the mosque. Ghazala still felt like herself, despite her difficulties, and got a deep sense of meaning from her faith. One day she might need to pray at home, as she wouldn't want to embarrass herself or her family, but Ghazala believed that, in helping her mother, Tahera would receive many blessings, and this was a great comfort to her.

The most important relationships for a continuing sense of self are with what gives each one of us a sense of meaning, which can be religion, nature, art or even our grandchildren. These connections are not dependent on cognitive abilities, spiritual experiences or our ability to talk to others about these. I know that I *experience* divine love, even if I can no longer *express* this experience clearly to others. My inability to describe my experiences of the divine does not mean that I do not have them, which underscores the importance of an insider's view to examining a continuing sense of self in dementia. My relationship with God 'is in no way compromised if grounded in neurological substrate...a graceful God remains present...to the very end' (Post 1998, p.211), and I continue to have the unique human capacity to relate to God and to others (Brown 2004, pp.67–68).

Despite living with dementia, we can experience a relationship with the divine, or with what gives us a sense of meaning. We might need support to get to the place where we can experience this connection, or help to practice any familiar rituals, but we are still able to have meaningful relationships that reach deep within, to what feels like the centre of our being. From my viewpoint, we 'know each other not as brains ensheathed in bodies but as embodied persons. We are people who relate to each other as beings created in the image of God' (Jones 2004, p.31), and can relate to what gives us a sense of meaning 'in a manner that reaches deeply into the essence of our creaturely, historical, and communal selves' (Brown 1998, p.101). This is the key to understanding the importance of relationships to us all, and how those that give us meaning can uplift us by reaching to the centre of our being.

We cannot lose our membership of humanity, nor our ability to relate to what gives us a sense of meaning, simply by losing our neurones. How can either our ability to respond in relationships with others, or to what gives us an inner sense of meaning, possibly be touched by damage to our brain? Being in relationships is an integral part of being human. If people with dementia are thought to be unable to be in relationships with others, or to find a sense of meaning in places such as worship spaces, in nature or through music or art, surely this casts them out from what it means to be human? Are we no longer part of human community? 'Human existence…is always lived out within human community… To be a person is to be a member of the human race' (Swinton 2012, p.156). Indeed, as my cognitive ability fades, I have felt a greater sense of emotional connection within the community, and an increasing relationship with the divine, and write, 'The scrambling of my cognitive and emotional abilities has not diminished my spirit, or my relationship with the divine' (Bryden 2016, p.14). Despite cognitive difficulties, I still have a sense of spiritual connection with the divine, through the familiar words spoken within the fellowship of my faith community.

I have gained great reassurance from placing my cognitive struggles in the context of a relationship with the divine, in stillness, despite my jumbled cognition. Surely our muddled thoughts, scrambled words and odd behaviours cannot mean that we have lost our ability to connect with what gives us meaning? We might need help to say the right words or do the right things but, in our hearts and spirits, we can depend on a continuing sense of self to relate to the divine, to nature or to what has always given us a sense of meaning.

Relating from birth

Dovu stood quietly in his living room, in front of the little statue of Buddha, and lit some incense, which was part of his daily ritual. He was determined to keep on doing this as long as he could, despite his decline due to dementia. He was finding it harder to work out how to light the matches, let alone manage the incense, but his wife, Mima, was helping him today, as she knew this was important to him. But Dovu was finding meditation particularly difficult, as his mind would wander all over the place, like a naughty monkey swinging amongst the branches high above the jungle. Mima could not help him here: his thoughts flittered about to and fro, leaping around with no rhyme or reason. How could he possibly concentrate and make his mind like a still mountain pool? How could he remain focused on his mind, body and feelings? Where had his mindfulness gone? It seemed even more elusive than it had ever been. However, Dovu had spoken to the master of his temple about all of this, who had talked about the sense of 'now' that Dovu seemed to be experiencing all of the time. This present moment was central to Dovu's experience of dementia; he couldn't recall the past, nor know what the future held, but felt as if he was treading water in the present time. His master had reassured Dovu that this was the essence of Buddhism, living in the present, where 'now' is the ground of all being. Maybe he was becoming a better Buddhist because of having dementia!

My embodied relational self is a way of being, not doing; I am part of the human family, relating to others from birth till death. Indeed, *we are all human beings, not human doings*. Before my diagnosis, I used to be asked what I did, and had an answer for such questions. These cognitive masks of my doings are being stripped away to reveal vital aspects of my sense of self, or of my being, that lie within. Far more important to me is who I am, and to know the relationships around me that give me comfort and a sense of support and encouragement. People with dementia are sometimes thought to lose our ability to relate to others, but how can that be? We can relate to others by eye contact, touch, a smile, and perhaps a few words, however muddled. We can communicate our needs, as well as our sense of pain, pleasure and concern.

Philosopher John Macmurray argues that the newborn relates to her mother and is able to communicate her needs from birth (1999, pp.48–50). My mother regarded me from the moment of my birth as an embodied relational self, never as an empty shell of a body until I had full capacities.

Surely, even with a fading cognitive capacity, I am still a fully embodied relational self, able to communicate my needs? When I was a baby, and now living with dementia, I could then, and will continue to be able to, express my needs in relationship until death. As Swinton points out, a mother *teaches* her baby such things as 'relationality, communication, identity and a...firm sense of self' (2014, p.242). She does not do this in order that her child becomes a human, but assumes that she is nurturing certain capacities in her infant, who is already a member of humanity. *Dementia cannot take this birthright away.*

We are all continuing embodied relational selves: 'from birth, we are in the process of becoming, and this "becoming" is encoded in our brains by means of synaptic activity as both nature and nurture...form and reform the developing self' (Green 2008, p.85). We all begin life as helpless infants, then we age and become dependent on others again: dependence and vulnerability are common to us all at the beginning and end of our lives. Ethicist John Wyatt writes in particular of the vulnerability of late life, when he describes how his mother had been transformed into dependency by dementia (2009, p.65).

We cannot regard human life as either emerging or disappearing; we are all continuing embodied relational selves, and this is not dependent at any stage in our lives on our ability to relate, remember or communicate. Babies are not humans in the making, *any more than I am a human in the unmaking*. This idea of potentiality, and of its loss, raises the question of why – or indeed when – should I lose my membership of the human family? This is a major concern for people with dementia, who, shockingly, can be regarded, as I have mentioned, as empty shells from whom the self has departed. We remain fully human at all stages in our journey with dementia, and we are never empty bodies devoid of self.

My relational self began in the form of meaningful images, such as the familiar face of my mother, as I perceived the world around me and distinguished myself from others and from my environment. Gradually I learnt words to label and store these images; then my family told stories about me, and through these stories I began to understand who I was, gaining a sense of being an embodied relational self. Now the experience of dementia is being included as part of the story of my unfolding life as this embodied relational self.

Capacities for relationship

Keith was a keen golf player, and had many friends at his local club. In order to make sure he could keep up his golf, despite increasing difficulties due to his dementia, his wife Angela had arranged for his colleagues to keep score, reassuring them that he was not cheating, but just getting muddled up with the numbers. She had also described other problems that Keith might have, with language and recall, as Angela was very much hoping that his friends would be continue to be faithful supporters for him. His golf meant a great deal to Keith, and he still wanted to keep on playing a game each week, repairing to the nineteenth hole with his friends after the game. It seemed as if, despite his problems in finding the right word now and then – let alone recalling his golf buddies' names – he could still find a place alongside them at the club. Keith was quite capable of relating to people, and was as friendly as always, asking people how they were – even if he could not recall their reply from moment to moment, day to day, or week to week. His smile was as broad as ever, and he was unfailingly polite and helpful. Keith still got a deep sense of meaning from nature, and his walk around the golf course gave him that connection with the greenery around him. He had never been particularly religious, but in a way his golf was his faith, and took him out into broad expanses of grass, under shady trees and beneath an ever-changing sky. Very importantly, it was also a way of connecting him with others who shared his love of golf, which was beyond words and complicated sentences. Keith felt supported in these friendly relationships and always came back feeling recharged, reinvigorated and refreshed.

Psychologist Warren Brown's view is that we have six enhanced capacities 'critical for personal relatedness' (1998, pp.103–104; my emphasis): language, theory of mind, episodic memory, conscious top-down agency, future orientation and emotional modulation. Brown's assumption is that these capacities diminish with increasing cognitive disability, and that the continuing relational self of people with dementia is at risk. How can an outsider such as Brown describe our experience of being in meaningful relationships? In the following, I write about each of these so-called enhanced critical capacities, in regard to people with dementia, and demonstrate that we retain the ability to relate to others.

Language

Brown's view is that language is essential in relationships, in order to convey complex ideas and concepts of the past and future (1998, p.103). This indeed could exclude *all* people with communication difficulties, as well as babies, let alone those with dementia! However, I can still relate to others, despite occasionally having to communicate *nonverbally* due to words failing me. Even those who have lost all language ability can still communicate through eye contact and facial expression – or indeed by the simple means of grasping a hand, such as that Japanese lady in Matsue I mentioned earlier.

Unlike many outside observers, Sabat makes a significant contribution towards seeing the world through our eyes, and is able to do this despite our communication problems. He is an expert in listening directly to the voice of people with dementia, conceiving of 'mind', or what I regard as self, as a process arising in discourse, akin to an internal conversation (Sabat 2001, p.222); this is what I call the embodied relational self. Sabat understands how communication difficulties can form a barrier to meaningful relationships, so that we feel imprisoned behind the barrier of language difficulties and recall dysfunction, yet we are still here as embodied relational selves. Swinton writes of the possibility that dementia 'locks people in' behind cognitive incapacity, and reflects on whether spirituality might be the key to unlock the person 'in the stillness of that spiritual moment' (2011, p.181). I do in fact often feel 'locked in' because of my muddled words and mixed up grammar, and so often I see my husband struggle to understand what I am saying. But, in the stillness of my relationship with him as a sympathetic other, I can be restored by the acceptance of my efforts at nonverbal communication.

I share some of the linguistic difficulties observed by Sabat; for example, Dr B. had interrupted attention and a subsequent shifted conversation flow, due to being unable to inhibit the processing of other sources of information when trying to communicate (Sabat 2001, p.53). I have written of 'crossed wires misfiring' (Bryden 2005, p.64), when my words become interrupted by visual or aural cues. Peculiar words then interrupt my sentences, so that an object that I am idly looking at can somehow become placed in a completely unrelated sentence, to make no sense whatsoever. For example, I could be talking to my husband about going shopping, and all the things we need, and then suddenly insert the word 'telephone' or 'tree' into my sentence!

Negative emotions can also further impede word finding, such as Dr M.'s anguish at her impaired language (Sabat 2001, p.73). I have similar feelings of despair at my inability to come up with the correct word, when I know that one exists. There is no way to find that word and there is no asking my husband; I wave my hands about anxiously, and words become increasingly misplaced and misspoken. In my writing and speaking this is becoming more and more frustrating, as my verbal skills are now becoming significantly diminished. Now it is taking an increasing amount of time for me to search around for the complex thoughts that might make this book a reality, and to find the words to express these ideas. I need to have patience with myself, when this was never a trait of mine!

Sabat's work is in contrast to the much earlier study of sociologist Jaber Gubrium, who interviewed care-partners, who expressed the view that was common around the time of my diagnosis: 'Hidden as it is, mind *must* be spoken for' (1986, p.43; my emphasis). However, the mind, or what I refer to as the self, need not be spoken for, as we are all dependent on the abilities of others to interact and connect with our social and independent selves (Swinton 2012, pp.60–62). We *all* assume that others have a self with which to perceive the world, and we try to imagine what others mean when they express themselves. People with dementia need others to give us the benefit of the doubt, and to assume that we have a self, and that we have views that we are trying to convey. Try to understand us, have patience and, importantly, *give us time.*

I have personal thoughts, ideas, images and concepts, which I might have difficulties expressing, due to word-finding problems, yet this is only one part of communication. We all communicate nonverbally, relying on others to see, as well as hear, what we are saying. In my talks, I say *listen with your eyes,* to suggest that care-partners should watch for this expressive form of communication (Bryden 2015b, p.215). Rather than saying that the mind is hidden, I suggest that the top third of the iceberg of communication, or our ability to find words, is indeed obscured. However, the two-thirds beneath the surface represents our nonverbal communication, and can be explored, as we struggle to communicate what we want to say.

Theory of mind

Theory of mind is the ability to attribute mental states to others, and to have an awareness of one's own mental state, so that to communicate effectively, humans need to be able to read the body language and intentions of others. People with dementia retain this ability, and are extremely sensitive, not necessarily to the words you use, but to how you say them. In my talks, I have often said that *it is not what you say, but how you say it that is important*. Watch for any nonverbal expression that may accompany your words, to which people with dementia will respond. We will attribute to others the mental state that this nonverbal expression represents, such as annoyance or apathy, rather than the actual words.

Brown writes of metacognition, or 'thinking about thinking', and makes assumptions that this ability is gradually lost in people with dementia, despite their lifetime of experiences (1998, p.108). This is an outsider's viewpoint and, although there has been considerable research on the development of metacognition in children, assumptions concerning its loss in people with dementia may well be incorrect. For example, intact social cognition is found amongst people with dementia, and with their care-workers (Sabat and Gladstone 2010, p.74). There appears to be a social cognition reserve in these adults, which has been developed over the course of their lives and is now retained throughout the experience of dementia.

Episodic memory

Brown proposes that episodic memory is vital to relating to others (1998, p.113), which of course would be problematic to people with dementia, as we do find it hard to recall past events. However, why should an accurate recall of the historical record of my life, and those of others', be essential in relationships? Although I cannot recall my recent history, nor a friend's name or her history, I can relate to her in the moment, without needing to use her name or to ask knowledgeably about happenings in her recent past. Even if I cannot recall her label, or what is attached to this label, I can still connect deeply moment to moment, where my relationships give me an important aspect of my sense of self.

Conscious top-down agency

Top-down agency is the ability to regulate behaviour in regard to conscious thought, as well as intentions (Brown 1998, p.103). This capacity has been shown to be retained in people with dementia (McFadden *et al.* 2000): elderly residents of a nursing home were active agents, engaging with their environments, with staff and with one another. They showed a wide range of emotions, including, importantly, a caring sensitivity for one another.

Sabat and Lee (2011) also observed social interactions in which there were interpersonal understandings amongst people with dementia, based on regulating their behaviour appropriately.

Future orientation and emotional modulation

Due to a disturbed sense of time and of recall, I cannot envisage future scenarios. Nor do I have reliable emotional modulation, as my reactions are less repressed than they used to be, so that I am more emotional in my responses. Brown regards both of these capacities as being vital to relatedness (1998, pp.103–104). However, I can listen to future scenarios, and reflect the feelings I am hearing. I am able to be present in the moment, and attend to feelings and emotions. Such *reflective listening* is a vital aspect for all of our relationships, and indeed forms the basis of successful counselling. My capacity to do this has not been diminished by my lived experience of dementia.

Summary

All of Brown's six criteria (1998, pp.103–104) are an *outsider's* view of human capacities for relationships. They imply that it is impossible to have a sense of being an embodied relational self, unless all six capacities are present. In my exploration of a continuing sense of self in the lived experience of dementia, I find that personal relatedness is not diminished by cognitive disability. I suggest that Brown's focus is on examining how humans might be superior to nonhuman species, rather than on how all humans might share in a capacity to relate to each other and to what gives them meaning in life, despite a range of disabilities.

Mind you, as a nonhuman species, our poodle certainly can show, from my own outsider's viewpoint, some of these capacities! He seems to be able to communicate nonverbally, or at least by facial expression, a bark or a whimper; he seems to recall things that are important to him, whether negative or positive, such as his favourite toy (joy!) or a visit to the vet (fear!); he seems to be able to show empathy with me when I feel stressed, and also seems to be able to read my mind, especially if that relates to a walk!

Nevertheless, Brown does point to the importance of 'being related to' by others, so that babies are included (1998, p.124). Therefore, surely people with dementia should also be included, even if our relatedness might require extra effort by others (p.125)? Indeed, we have an increasing dependence on others, as we become less able to do as much as we might want. I rely on my enabler, my husband, to help me to do what I can, while I can. However, this can result in a fine balance, as we do not want others to do everything for us, as then we can be at risk: care-partners or enablers can 'smother us with care…[and we] fade as we withdraw from trying' (Bryden 2015b, p.80). This can impact negatively and result in 'excess disability' (Sabat 2001, p.94), where we are far less capable than we might be, due to a lack of practice. It is increasingly important for us to keep on trying to do things, as we can very rapidly forget our skills.

Our personality, character and how others see us should not be placed at risk, as this can result in negative positioning of people with dementia in social encounters (Swinton 2012, p.89), in which we are stripped of all other descriptors of our lives. For example, I do not want to be introduced in social situations as a person with dementia. I am so much more: a wife, mother, grandmother, author and researcher! I write, 'Maintain our dignity and avoid depersonalizing us' (Bryden 2015b, p.224).

8

Narrative self

Mary had been living with dementia for a year or so now. She wasn't sure how long, but it felt as if she had always had that label attached to her, and she didn't like it one bit! She still loved her garden, and she had just planted some beautiful flowers and was looking forward to seeing them grow and blossom. Mary had 'green fingers' – it was part of who she was. But would she always have this ability and, more importantly, would she know she had this ability? Would she still be able to potter in her garden? Of course, as she grew older and frailer, it might become physically more problematic, but she hoped with all of her heart that she could always enjoy her flowers, even if it was just in pots on a patio or balcony. Her flowers gave her a sense of meaning, and were part of who she was. Everyone knew of her flowers – who would Mary be without her splendid array of her favourite blossoms? What really worried her was whether she would lose her story, and all that gave her meaning in life – not just her flowers. She wondered if she would recall her marriage, children, grandchildren, and all her happy holidays with her lovely husband. What would this mean – would she then be just a vegetable without a story? However, her grandchildren were a great source of delight and gave her such joy. They never seemed to mind her difficulties in remembering all their names or their stories – she could relate to them in the moment and hoped this would continue.

The question in many people's minds is whether dementia might strip us of our story. It is what people fear most – a loss of an autobiography, or a narrative of our life. Narrativity is described as a 'human-forming, meaning-making enterprise' (Green 2008, p.121), and as being 'part of our survival toolkit' (Bryan 2016, p.53). We gain a sense of who we are by virtue of our story. However, I do not agree that 'for human beings stories are an essential part of our *cognitive* architecture' (Bryan 2016, p.29; my emphasis), as I can still explore meaning, beyond a limited cognitive timeline of events, towards a richer expression of all that I am. Despite fading cognition, I continue to be a narrative self who is able to find meaning and a sense of identity *in the present moment*. Why should an accurate recall of a series of past events mean so much in finding out who we are as a person, or what gives us a sense of meaning in life? As I wrote before, a robot could be programmed to recall all the events in its so-called 'life', yet it cannot be regarded to know what it is, let alone have a sense of meaning!

I cannot tell you reliably a series of past events in my life, without my husband's or daughters' help. It has faded into a muddle, and even if I am helped to recall something, it is not always clear. I might not always recall being there, even if I am told that this is what I did and where I was. I no longer always seem to have that clear video record of my life, and often have only the words of others who are trying to prompt my recall. Yet, despite the lack of a remembered precise chronological record, I still have 'a concept of self whose unity resides in the unity of a narrative which links birth to life to death as narrative beginning to middle to end' (MacIntyre 1981, p.91). I have a continuing sense of self, as a thread connecting me to my past and to my future, even if it is broken and reliant on the assistance of others. Sometimes it feels as if the beautiful pearl necklace of my life has broken, the gems are being scattered, and I am asking for help trying to re-thread them into some sort of order again!

Surely, recall dysfunction, an unreliable sense of time and language difficulties do not mean that I no longer have a coherent narrative? Despite disease and frailty, we all have and are a meaningful story, where 'our journey through life is a continuing one of assigning meaning, reviewing meaning, and reframing our own narrative' (MacKinlay 2016, p.33). My life still has meaning, even with dementia, which is mine to 'learn how to read and interpret' (Swinton 2012, p.164).

Recall and narrative

The common view that recall dysfunction means a loss of self, and that a person thereby no longer has a meaningful narrative, can be traced back to Plato and Aristotle, who had a simple view of recall as being similar to modern data storage and retrieval (Keck 1996, p.64). Like that robot I mentioned earlier, having a meaningful narrative would mean a series of events stored in the motherboard! Saint Augustine was also influential in regard to ideas of recall, and writes, 'It is I myself who remembers, I the mind' (Augustine 1996, p.265). This focus on the mind, or the 'I' being the thing that remembers, appears to imply that people with dementia, whose recall is impaired, have no sense of being an 'I' or have no sense of self. These views of our mind, our 'I' or our self being reliant on accurate recall of all past events still persist, yet almost no one has this type of photographic recall from which to create a sense of narrative self. Very few people can recall a conversation in the past in any great detail, or an event in their childhood with any particular clarity, and are then able to relate this to others with great confidence as an absolutely correct historical record.

Theologian Peter Kevern appears to share the common outsider's view of recall dysfunction: that it leads to a loss of 'meaning and emotional connection. We are narrated creatures, and as the narrative is interrupted, so we sense our very being becoming incoherent and intermittent' (2012, p.48). *How would he know*, if he has not experienced a problematic recall? Even with my disrupted recall, and my need for help to reconstruct past events, I still feel as if I have a history and an unbroken thread of existence as an embodied relational self. Other outsiders also suggest that I *must* be able to sequence events in time in order to create meaning, which implies that a remembered chronology is vital to having and being a story (Baldwin and Estey 2015, p.216).

These are outsiders' views of my narrative becoming disrupted as a consequence of my recall dysfunction. They assume that my narrative is reliant on having an accurate recall of events on my timeline but, without help, I am unable to recall such events today, or in the past few days, weeks, months or recent years. Despite a lack of precise recall, I can still write this book and reflect on meaning. I do not consider that my remembered history is critical, as *I am who I am now, and meaning is what I can find in this present moment*. My narrative results from finding meaning in life and developing a sense of identity in the present moment, not based on events in the past.

Language and narrative

Language is not critical for me to *be* a story, although to *share* my narrative I may need to be helped. Therefore I do not agree that narrative 'brings experience into language' (Baars 2012, p.155), as I can still have and be a story despite my linguistic problems. My own experiences and observations of people in the later stages of dementia support Damasio's idea of a *nonverbal narrative*, dependent on the coordination of deep brain structures, where the autobiographical 'self comes to mind in the form of images, relentlessly telling a story of such engagements' (2010, p.203). I still have this stream of images depicting my narrative, despite difficulties in finding the right descriptors, or in sorting these pictures into accurate order. Therefore, I am still able to find a personal sense of meaning in life, and develop a sense of identity, even in the form of imagery, despite language loss.

Present moment and narrative

Recall dysfunction has given me a new relationship with time, so that I feel situated in the present, no longer able to recall the past. However, I am still a historical being, who lives in time, and my narrative conveys 'what it is to live in the world or in worlds, but also what it *means* to live in time' (Baars 2012, p.150). I continue to be a story in my world and in the relationships and environment around me (Baars 2012, p.161). I agree with Eastern Orthodox theologian John Zizoulas that a 'capacity for memory is not necessarily a unique characteristic' of self, nor is needed for me to have and be a narrative (Zizoulas 1975, pp.416–417).

Reflecting on my narrative in a process of making meaning involves feelings and emotions, as well as my sense of the present moment. Episodes in my life exist 'in a tensed temporal modality; both past and future are inseparable from lived present experience' (Bryan 2016, p.27). This modality is like Sabat's 'personal present' (Sabat 2001, p.232), within which a fear of future possibilities, as well as an awareness of my past, reshaped my narrative shortly after diagnosis, and continue to influence my search for meaning. Fears of future loss, as well as struggles with ongoing decline, impact negatively on my personal present. However, my present moment is filled with many other aspects of my life and, within this abundance, my sense of self can continue to flourish.

An inability to recall cognitive facts, and having a disturbed sense of time, does not impact on our ability to find meaning in life, so that people with dementia can continue to develop a sense of meaning in the present moment. Spiritual reminiscence work with people with dementia has shown that meaning can be found in the moment, where narrative is still possible for people with dementia (MacKinlay and Trevitt 2012, pp.16–17). Sabat also writes that the people with dementia he worked with were able to make and derive meaning in the present moment (2001, p.160), similar to my goals in this book. I can find purpose and unity in life, 'creating a coherent, meaningful spiritual self-story' in which I transcend self, not by separating from but by connecting to others and to what gives me a sense of meaning (Poll and Smith 2003, p.139).

9

Upheld by Others in the Fullness of Our Identity

Recently diagnosed with dementia, Susan was terrified of the future, and felt overwhelmed by what she might face. Her family lived far away, and it was easy to simply say everything was fine when they rang to see how she was. But, as a devout Catholic, how could she possibly find any meaning in this experience of dementia? She felt confused most days, and could not recall people's names, or even what had happened in their lives. She had to rely on others to connect with her and to give her a bit of leeway for not being sympathetic or congratulatory when this was due. Susan began to feel like a bad person for not being a good friend anymore. Where was God in all of this – where was there any meaning in having dementia? Had God abandoned her? It felt like an overwhelming tragedy, yet her church community surrounded her with love, making her casseroles, giving her lifts, and ringing her to check that she was OK. Someone always took her to Mass, even though she found it was hard sometimes to do the right things during the worship. However, she drank in the sights, sounds, and smells – the familiarity of the Mass where she had always found a deep sense of meaning – and gained a feeling of inner peace.

I am so much more than my recall dysfunction, disrupted sense of time and communication problems: even if I can no longer speak, and my thoughts become more muddled, I will have a continuing sense of meaning – a continuing sense of being an embodied relational self. In writing of narrative loss, when recall of events fades, Swinton poses the question: 'Who will tell our stories well when we have forgotten who we are?' (2012, p.23). However, I suggest that we do not forget who we are, but that we do need help to uncover a narrative of meaning in the present moment, in which can be found many aspects of our story. Keck writes that 'we are also what others remember of us' (1996, p.43), and Swinton further develops this concept, writing that 'we are not what we remember; we are remembered' (2012, p.198). Indeed, our family and friends have memories of us, and all these various memories add up to a broad perspective of the many facets of our nature. We are remembered even after we die, leaving a legacy in the lives of those left behind.

Dementia might be tragic, but so is the human condition – ultimately the outcome of all human life is decay and death (Swinton 2012, pp.184–185). I believe that others can uphold us as we travel this journey with dementia, helping us to find meaning despite what might seem like an apparent hopelessness. We can find and treasure moments of joy, moments when we connect to what gives us a sense of meaning, and moments when we feel surrounded by others in relationships of love and acceptance. In particular, focusing on the present moment is of great value to us, where we can find the transcendence that resonates with an experience of sharing from a sense of 'now', when we are far more than our ability to recall; we are able to find and share a sense of meaning.

I am inspired by the story of Jimmie, whose recall dysfunction was so severe that neurologist Oliver Sacks thought of him as having no spirituality (Sacks 1985, p.36). However, in chapel, he observed Jimmie's experience of 'continuity and reality, in the absoluteness of spiritual attention and act' and that 'there remains the undiminished possibility of reintegration by art, by communion, by touching the human spirit: and this can be preserved in what seems at first a hopeless state of neurological devastation' (1985, pp.37–38). Like Jimmie, my sense of the numinous gives me great hope and meaning in the present moment, despite my cognitive difficulties.

My narrative continues to be formed and reformed in embodied relationships within the community, where we are all 'living narratives' (Bryan 2016, p.44). I still am and have a meaningful story, even though my language and recall are impaired. Although I have a diminishing ability to express this unfolding narrative of meaning, it does not mean that I do not experience it: 'my life is like a carpet unrolling before and behind me' (Bryden 2015b, p.130). In this metaphor, life before and behind me is unseen, yet the pattern of meaning beneath my feet is nonetheless vivid, although I might need more help and time to describe it.

My functioning on neuropsychological tests is becoming increasingly defective, yet these do not measure my sense of embodied relational self, nor my ability to find meaning in the present moment. I can still explore my fears of loss and develop the concept of having a sense of being an embodied self in relationships. My published work has been a process of finding meaning, which is furthered in this book, as I challenge the story of loss of self in dementia with an insider's perspective.

We need to be supported in an inclusive community of equals

Mark had been diagnosed many years ago now, and was losing much of his ability to talk and to recall things about his past. He had lost many of his friends now, but he could still smile and chat in the moment with those around him. He loved the Masonic Lodge, where he had been going for years. The rituals were familiar and it was a splendid place, where his wife, Kay, was now quite important. Here everyone accepted him as an equal, maybe remembering him in his past roles? But at church, it seemed to be very different. Kay was concerned to see Mark sitting alone in one of the front pews, where they always sat, because she was up at the front doing the readings. It was such as shame that no one seemed to sit with him or talk to him any more. After the service Mark used to be able to chat with everyone, often talking of his time with a major company and his successful career. Now he was nearly always left alone to sit at a table, until Kay came alongside him to make the conversation flow easily. Kay wished that church was as welcoming as the Lodge, and that people would simply sit with Mark and accept him as he was. Why couldn't it be a place of welcome, as it should be if it was to follow what was in the gospel? Surely everyone, no matter what his or her ability to chat or recall, should be welcomed in church?

For people with dementia to be supported in the community, a *communal* form of relatedness is vital, as this can enfold us all as equals. Our communities need to include all people, despite their varying physical and cognitive capacities. 'As persons in relation, we are called…into community where the weak and the strong, the insightful and the forgetful flourish together' (Hudson 2016, p.65). In suggesting communal relatedness for our communities, I have examined theologian Martin Buber's concept of 'I–You', which is an extensive exploration of the nature of *individual* relationships, both interpersonal and objective, focusing on the 'I' of the I–You and I–It (Buber 1937/1970, p.54). However, I do not feel that this model of individual relationship can offer an adequate template for inclusive communities. As Kevern writes, 'we do not hold our identities as individuals, but as members of communities' (2012, p.48). We need to be liberated from the concept of cognitive function being necessary for participating in a community of people, and allow for gatherings of people of *all varying physical and cognitive capacities.*

We need to move towards a *collective identity*, which might be difficult for our modern society to appreciate, but Eastern Orthodox tradition is helpful, as it views 'individuality as a perversion' (Zizoulas 1975, p.441). It is hard for people with dementia to participate in a post-modern community that measures people on the basis of their cognition, as we cannot demonstrate the autonomy and intellect that is required. However, we would be able to participate more freely in inclusive and diverse communities, where we were accepted as part of a collective identity.

The concept of individual autonomy is a characteristic of modern times, and theologian Stanley Grenz discusses how this first arose with Saint Augustine, who was looking for an inner self (Grenz 2006, pp.71–77). Individuality is rarely seen in the ancient Middle East, where well-defined personal boundaries were less important than living in community: 'men and women experienced personal identity as they lived in community with other persons' (Weaver 1986, p.447). As biblical scholar Joel Green points out, in these times, people could not 'be understood in their individuality' (1998, p.158); even those who played a prominent role remained embedded within the community.

Little children, as well as people with dementia, can be included within collective communities. It seems obvious that children should not be excluded, for at what stage do they become fully human? Surely, I should also be included, for at what stage do I become no longer human? Instead of society's perception of my diminishing capacity, such a community can emphasise equality, and include me as an equal.

How can the community support and include us?

My circle of friends diminished after diagnosis, probably due to their fears of whether I could behave in socially accepted ways. Now, with increasing recall dysfunction, I forget that my friends exist and what is happening in their lives, so I am more dependent on my friends to continue to relate to and remember me. However, people cannot be forced to, or embarrassed into, being my friends, so a change in their hearts is needed; the best way to do this is to 'put yourself in my shoes' (Bryden 2015b, p.201). I seek to be supported within an inclusive community that emphasises diversity, rather than cognition, where I can be welcomed as an equal.

By 'casting off the straitjacket' of society's views of loss, a diverse community can include people with dementia and regard them as having a continuing sense of self, including a sense of meaning in the present moment. Can this be a remembering community and help me to keep my story safe? Can it relate to me and respect me, despite my impairments? I might be less able to be defined by my sense of cognitive self; however, I continue to be an embodied relational self with a narrative of meaning in the present moment, who seeks to belong, be welcomed and be shown hospitality. I am still 'me' to whom my friends can relate, and what I need is for the community to remember that my life has meaning, just as I am, despite my dementia. Can the community 'hear others into speech and assist in the re-patterning of broken and fragmented lives' (Walton 2002, p.3)?

Society fears dementia and we can become isolated, as people do not how to relate to us, nor what to say. Yet, in an inclusive community, we can see beyond our differences, towards appreciating humanity in all of its diversity. There is no difference between us: I am part of our common existence in the fullness and diversity of humanity. We all have many differences: physical and cognitive ability, looks and many other aspects of our lives, yet we are all part of the richness of human life.

People with dementia may look familiar, but we are changing, so that we find it hard to meet the community's expectations of polite and so-called normal behaviour. These changes can result in us becoming isolated, pushed towards the margins of society, where we are becoming like strangers. However, we need others to include us in the community despite our difficulties; not out of pity or out of duty, but knowing we are all equal within humanity's rich diversity. We need to be welcomed in friendship, and missed when we have not been seen for a while. By *offering us a welcome with delight,* this can overcome the power of dementia to isolate us: say, 'It's good that you exist; it's good that you are in this world!' (Kinghorn 2016, p.112.) This type of welcome makes us feel as if we belong, which is so much more than simply being included. Inclusion would mean the community simply tolerates our presence, rather than welcoming us with delight.

People with dementia are 'like outcasts in today's hyper-cognitive society' (Bryden 2015b, p.287). Unfortunately, some people stop relating to us, perhaps because we have forgotten who they are, and they want to be remembered. Unfortunately, they may even stop visiting us, as we might not remember previous visits, or their name and how they relate to us. However, we will respond in the moment to the emotion and warmth of a visit (Bryden 2015b, p.133):

> Your name, the label that belongs to you, often is not there. Your face is familiar somehow, but meeting you happens too quickly for me to search through my disjointed memory and find a label for you... Don't just give me your label, as I need more than that to really know who you are... The way I know people is in a spiritual and emotional way. There's a knowing of who a person is right at their core. But I have no idea who they are, in terms of who they are meant to be in your world, of cognition and action, and labels and achievement... Why must I remember who you are? Is this just to satisfy your own need for identity? Your visit is not a cognitive experience that I will store and recall. Let me live in the present. (Bryden 2005, pp.109–110)

We might seem odd due to our cognitive decline and increasing strangeness, but there can be no 'us' and 'them' in an inclusive and diverse community, in which we seek relationships that recognise our difficulties. We find it hard to communicate, as well as to follow what is said, and respond quickly enough. These can seem like insurmountable problems for others, but we need to be given '*cognitive ramps*' (Bryden 2015b, p.214; my emphasis). Sabat is very skilled in this regard, and accommodates linguistic difficulties, as well as long pauses, bridging the gap of these problems by taking what he calls 'the intentional stance' (Sabat 2001, p.37). Sabat searches for meaning in 'extra-linguistic communication such as tone of voice, facial expression, gesture' (p.217). Similarly, we need slower communication, allowing for pauses, and looking for meaning in nonverbal as well as verbal expression (Bryden 2015b, p.286). Post uses a different term for bridging these communicative difficulties, writing of '*prostheses*, filling in the gaps and expecting that now and then the cues we provide will connect with the person' (Post 2006, p.229; my emphasis). For example, I need such cues or prompts: instead of saying 'Wasn't it lovely yesterday?' say 'Wasn't it lovely yesterday, when we went for a picnic to the park, and you wore that dress with sunflowers?' I want my friends to keep going with such prompts, until they see the light in my eyes that means that I recall something from this event.

I live without a sense of time, so need to be accepted without an awareness of the hours or days passing. Theologian Jean Vanier spoke of being a '*friend of time*' when writing about the tensions of life in the L'Arche community for people with disabilities (Vanier 1979, p.89). People can come alongside me in my present moment, and be a friend of time; sitting with me in silence, using gesture, touch and eye contact in a language of listening. Swinton's description of this as 'the sacrament of the present moment' speaks to me of its nature as a meeting of spirit to spirit (2012, p.235). Part of coming alongside us is entering into our reality: 'Be imaginative, be creative, try to step across the divide between our worlds' (Bryden 2005, p.148). Post takes a similar view, writing, 'We are not obliged to reorient them into our reality, but we are obliged to be an attentive presence in theirs' (2004, p.14).

An inclusive community can hold our story faithfully, and challenge stories of loss in dementia with the view that we continue to have a sense of being an embodied self in relationships with others. MacKinlay highlights the importance of this role: 'it doesn't matter whether people can carry relevant memories themselves, but it does matter that other members of the body can carry those memories within a loving community' (2016, p.35). The community needs to counter negative stories of loss in dementia and, in so doing, should use Alzheimer's Australia's language guidelines (Alzheimer's Australia n.d.). These guidelines are referred to globally for how to speak to us, about us and about our care-partners, as well as about our condition. 'Language has great power to tear down or to lift up – to demean us or to encourage us' and 'There is so much you can change in our lives simply by taking care about how you speak to us and about us' (Bryden 2015b, pp.208, 230).

The community plays a crucial role in offering support and care, and should uphold us within an 'attentive community of memory and hope' (Swinton 2012, p.223). We face a gradual decline in function until death, yet may spend many years in the community, where our humanity can be affirmed as we 'approach the end of life, when it is important to reflect, find a sense of meaning and nourish our spirit' (Bryden 2015b, p.190). We need to be enabled to bring meaning to our experience, such as through spiritual reminiscence (MacKinlay and Trevitt 2012, p.273), and be helped to find ultimate meaning:

> It's about being with us and connecting with us without words. Heal us by your presence – bring us peace – as you connect with our spirit deep within.
>
> Try to find out more about us, so you can help us to find meaning in our lives. Our life story is a springboard for meaningful engagement. You can carry our story for us and relate to us as a whole human being, with dignity and respect. Focus on what we can still do, rather than all the many things we can no longer do…
>
> Try to discard temporarily your own masks of cognition and emotion, so that you too can be truly present in the spirit, able to connect without words. Use touch, eye contact, music and aroma, and try to breach the barrier of communication between us. Look into our eyes and look for that spark that may alight when you connect. You are creating within us a moment of wellbeing. (Bryden 2015b, p.288)

Within my lived experience of dementia, I am still part of the diversity of humanity, and our common vulnerability in community. I may not be able to take an active part in all community activities, but I can still receive the gift of friendship in an inclusive community that emphasises our diverse humanity.

10

Who Am I Now If I No Longer Have Dementia?

Ellen was coping OK with having dementia, and was keeping herself busy. After the initial shock of the diagnosis, and having to stop work and move to a more affordable house, she was finding meaningful things to do. Much of what she was doing related to the Alzheimer's Association, and she would go to their events, speak at conferences, and try to encourage others going through this diagnosis process. Ellen had been divorced some years ago, but had two lovely daughters, who had been terribly upset by her diagnosis. But now they were all coming to terms with it, and family gatherings seemed back to normal. Ellen loved her grandchildren dearly, even though it was hard to cope with the noisy boisterous boys when they stayed overnight. This dementia seemed to have taken away her ability to cope with more than one thing at a time, and certainly had impacted on her ability to cope as a grandmother for any longer than one night's stay. It had been a few years now, and she was going back to her specialist for her regular check-up, having had yet more tests and scans. Ellen sat in the specialist's rooms as the doctor walked in, with a big smile on her face. What was that about? The specialist calmly told Ellen that she didn't have dementia after all, and that it was Lyme's disease, which could be cured by an extended course of antibiotics. She then asked where Ellen might have been to catch Lyme's disease. Ellen just felt frozen to the spot, and couldn't think. She had no answers. How could she possibly not have dementia any more, after all that she had been through? This was awful – what about having given up work, moved house, and coping with a much smaller income? What about all those talks she had given and how public she had been about her experiences with dementia? How would her family cope with another huge upset in their lives?

Re-diagnosis is perhaps far more common than we realise; I have had several friends who have gone through this awful experience. As if the initial diagnosis was not shocking enough, this is even more traumatic! One woman was indeed told that her symptoms had been due to Lyme's disease; yet she had gone to international conferences to talk about having dementia and now needed to re-think who she was and what she should do in the future. Another was told that her symptoms were the result of chronic obstructive pulmonary disease; similarly, she had gone to several national conferences to talk about her experiences with dementia. What would she say now? Another woman was told that her symptoms were due to post-traumatic stress disorder and that, with some years of treatment, she should recover. These women had each undergone major changes in their lives after the their initial diagnosis; giving up work, moving house, and managing on much lower incomes. They had also been very public, speaking at events, helping to run support groups, and trying to encourage others.

At a recent meeting, a clinician from a memory clinic said proudly that much of its work was the re-diagnosing of patients. Somehow, we are meant to be ecstatic that we no longer have dementia! There is no insight into how this might feel after years of adjusting to what is a traumatic diagnosis, especially if we have been active in trying to reach out to others, speaking out or offering support. We feel totally in shock, and it feels almost as traumatic as the initial diagnosis; yet little support is offered to us at this time. We cannot respond with any pleasure, as all we can think about is the needless major changes that we have made in our lives. If only the first diagnosis were made more carefully to start with, so that we did not have to risk a second major adjustment on our journey of life!

A major question looms large for the person who once thought that they had dementia: *who are they now, and who will they be?* Their whole family needs to face major adjustments to this change of identity, and explanations need to be found for the symptoms that the person has experienced, and often continues to experience.

11

Conclusion

About a year after I was diagnosed, I began to visit people with dementia at a nearby care home, hoping to be able to connect with them, as well as find out more about what I had been told would face me in the years ahead. I used to pop in every few weeks or so, and on one of my visits I was asked by staff to visit Sarah; her family had asked someone to pray with her and perhaps to find out if she still had some semblance of her faith. Sarah had been a devout Christian all her life, but had been unable to talk for at least six months now, so her family were not sure what remained of her faith. As I opened her door and went into her room, I could see Sarah lying in a foetal position, under a cotton cellular blanket. She was very thin, her skin looked almost translucent, and I could see her breathing gently and steadily, seemingly at peace. So I sat beside her bed, touched her delicate hand very gently, praying quietly, and chose a suitable passage of scripture to read. One day, I went into the home, and was about to go to Sarah's room to visit her as usual, but the staff said that she had died. However, her family had wanted to let me know that, just a few days before her death, Sarah had said a few words to them that made it clear that she still had a deep faith. This clearly had given the family a deep sense of comfort, and they were very grateful for my faithful visiting. For me, this too was of great comfort, as it spoke to me of how, even at the last stages of dementia, when a person no longer seemed to be there, still he or she was listening, aware and drinking in deeply each one of your words. Sarah, despite all outward appearances, was not deaf. She had still been an embodied relational self who could relate to what gave her meaning in life, as well as have a narrative of meaning in the present moment. I felt uplifted; despite what others might say would lie ahead of me, I felt sure that even at the very last stages of my journey with dementia, like Sarah, I too would still be me, hearing you.

I was diagnosed with dementia in 1995, over 20 years ago now. Can you imagine what it must feel like to be told you have dementia, while being surrounded by assumptions of loss of self, and even to believe them yourself? Would my family be facing my 'departure' and if so, where would I be going? Would I really be leaving an empty shell behind? This idea that we might lose our self due to dementia overwhelms us at the time of diagnosis, and we feel oppressed by the surrounding view of society that such loss is what faces us now, or at some time in the future. These views have an extremely negative impact on those of us being diagnosed with dementia, and cannot be underestimated; they result in a paralysing fear. We wonder if, and when, we will experience a future loss of self. Everything we do or say is viewed through the prism (or is that 'prison'?) of dementia.

These negative views of dementia prompted my published work, which forms a portfolio of autobiographic narratives, exploring the lived experience. In this book, I have reflected on a key theme emerging in my work: the loss of self in dementia. By offering an *insider's* perspective, my aim is to encourage society to see people with dementia with new eyes, as having a continuing sense of being an embodied self in relationships to others and with what gives them a sense of meaning, as well as having a narrative of meaning in the present moment. I challenge the *outsider's* view of loss of self in dementia with an insider's perspective, proposing that three aspects of a sense of self are retained throughout the lived experience:

Embodied self: an aspect of my self that gives me my sense of being embodied as an 'I' with first-person feelings about the world around me, distinguishing self from non-self.

Relational self: an aspect of my self that gives me my sense of being an embodied self in relationships with others, and with what gives me meaning.

Narrative self: an aspect of my self that is able to find meaning in life and to develop a sense of narrative identity in the present moment.

Society values competence, intelligence and autonomy, and devalues those of us who might be unable to demonstrate these attributes. Assumptions are made about our lack of capability, and that we will eventually become a terrible burden for our care-partners. Dementia is accompanied by stigma, and everyone becomes awkward around us because they fear that we might show embarrassing behaviours. It is important to challenge these views of loss of self in dementia, which lead to stigma, isolation and fears of the future, in order to give people being diagnosed (and their families) hope for the present and into the future. My aim is to project a new world of possibility, so as to encourage society to respond in improved understanding, support and care for people with dementia.

I still feel very much 'me' and often say, 'I'm still here'! I now fully accept my life with dementia, and do as much as I can, while I can, to reach out and help others by speaking and writing about what I am learning along the way. However, I am not living in some 'make-believe' land, as I struggle to cope most days, finding language, way-finding and recall increasingly problematic. I am declining steadily, but although my sense of time, recall and language are gradually becoming more impaired, I can still explore my continuing sense of self. I grapple for words just out of reach; I struggle with many daily tasks, but I am still Christine, who can search for meaning within her lived experience of dementia. Why should problems with recall, sense of time or language diminish a sense of self? I continue to be 'me' and to see the world through 'my' eyes, in the present moment. I know that I am the same self who existed a while ago: even if I cannot remember the facts or feelings of what I did or felt at that time, this does not mean that I have lost a sense of self. I am able to have a sense of embodiment, be in relationships and find meaning. I can explore my lived experience in the present moment, and reflect on my unfolding narrative to discover a continuing sense of self, within my changing experiences of, and interactions with, the world.

The question in many people's minds is whether dementia might strip us of our story, and this is what people fear most – a loss of an autobiography or a narrative of our life. Despite fading cognition, I continue to be a narrative self who is able to find meaning and a sense of identity *in the present moment*. Although I have a diminishing ability to tell others about my unfolding narrative of meaning, it does not mean that I do not experience it. Despite a lack of precise recall, I can still write this book and reflect on meaning, where what is important is who I am now, and where meaning is what I can find in this present moment. This moment is filled with many aspects of my life and, within this abundance, my sense of self can continue to flourish. However, we might need help from others to treasure moments of joy, moments when we connect with what gives us a sense of meaning, and moments when we feel surrounded by relationships of love and acceptance. I still am and have a meaningful story, even though my language and recall are impaired.

Writing a book is not at all easy at the best of times; now there are increasing challenges due to my lived experience of dementia. These make the process of writing and analysis more difficult, yet at the same time more authentic, because they give insight into my sense of self as someone living with dementia. I live with dementia, and can reflect both about and from within these difficulties to delve deeper into meaning. Although the common view of dementia would question my ability to do this, with many arguing that a loss of sense of self occurs at some time during the lived experience, I am still able to examine my published work, refer to relevant literature, and reflect on the meaning of my ongoing experience in the present moment.

I can bear witness to my own experience of coping with a traumatic diagnosis, as well as attesting to the many stories of others who are living with dementia and continue to live their lives full of meaning. How could someone who does not have dementia explore the sense of self within the lived experience? However, I was once an outsider before my diagnosis, and believed the usual view of loss of self in dementia. It was this belief in future loss of self that made the diagnosis more traumatic, as I feared that I would indeed experience this at some time. Importantly, therefore, I can look at loss of self in dementia from both points of view.

I am experiencing the world differently as my cognition declines, but who am I as a physical, emotional and spiritual being examining various aspects of my self in this context? Although I am interacting with the world from an altered perspective, still my sense of self remains. I am not simply a bundle of attributes; there is much more to my life, my relationships and my sense of unity, which is shaping my personal identity. I am far more than a deteriorating self in an increasingly empty shell of a body, with disappearing neurones and neuronal pathways.

My cognitive abilities might be decreasing, yet I continue to have a sense of embodiment, in relationships with others and with what gives me meaning. I am the self, knower, subject and agent for my thoughts, which occur in relationships with others around me, and there has been no disruption to my sense of self at any time since diagnosis. By examining my changing perceptions since diagnosis, and finding new sources of meaning, I consider that people with dementia retain a sense of being embodied relational selves, with a narrative of meaning in the present moment.

Let me liken my sense of being an *embodied relational self* to a can of baked beans, which is gradually losing its label (my ability to relate effectively to others). At what stage will my metaphorical can of baked beans be so defective in having lost its label that it will have lost its 'baked bean-ness'? Surely, it will always be a can of baked beans, even if the label is totally stripped away? No matter how little communication or recall ability I have left, I remain an embodied relational self within the community. My 'baked beans' analogy may seem ridiculous, but no more so than the logical consequence of any idea that loss of communication and increasing recall dysfunction might mean loss of self.

I may be less able to be defined by my *doing*, but I will always remain an intact *being*, who needs to belong, to be related to, and to be included. We can still relate to others, despite often having to communicate *nonverbally* due to words failing us. We all communicate nonverbally, through facial expression and gestures and eye contact; people with dementia can still communicate in this way. Try to understand us, have patience and, importantly, *give us time*.

Everyone communicates nonverbally to some extent, and this is increasingly the case for those with limited language abilities. Therefore, *listen with your eyes!*

The most important aspect of my continuing sense of self is that which gives me a sense of meaning, which is not dependent on my cognitive abilities, my experiences or, importantly, my ability to talk about these. I know that I *experience* a sense of meaning, even if I can no longer *express* this experience clearly to others, which underscores the importance of an insider's view for examining a continuing sense of self in dementia. We are all embodied selves who relate to one another as an 'I' and recognise an 'I'.

I cannot lose my membership of humanity, nor my ability to relate to others, simply by losing my neurones. Being in relationships is an integral part of being human. If people with dementia are thought to be unable to be in relationships with others, surely this casts them out from what it means to be human? Are we no longer part of the human community? I am part of the human family, relating to others from birth till death. Indeed, *we are all human beings, not human doings.* Dementia cannot take this birthright away. We all begin life as helpless infants, then we age and become dependent on others again, where dependence and vulnerability are common to us all at the beginning and end of our lives. We cannot regard human life as either emerging or disappearing; we are all continuing embodied relational selves, and this is not dependent at any stage in our lives on our ability to relate, remember or communicate. Babies are not humans in the making, *anymore than I am a human in the unmaking.*

Even if I am less able to participate as part of the life of the community, I am a witness to what it means to be human: simply to be, rather than to do.

Language is not critical for me to *be* a story, although to *share* my narrative with others I may need to be helped. Outsiders' views assume that finding meaning is reliant on having an accurate recall of events on a timeline, yet we all have and are a meaningful story. Indeed, as I have suggested: a robot could be programmed to recall accurately the entire record of its 'life', yet it cannot be regarded to know what it is, or to have a sense of meaning. I wonder why a lack of a remembered timeline is so important to outsiders, who then regard me as having 'lost my self'?

My aim is to encourage society to look beyond the dominant story of loss of self in dementia, so that people of all varying cognitive and physical capacities can be included and welcomed. I seek to transform society's views, towards accepting that there is a continuing sense of self throughout the lived experience of dementia, so that people with dementia and their families can be better supported in our communities. I look to a future in which those of us who have difficulties in today's fast-paced world can be included as equals, where what is important is who we are, not what we do. We seek to be welcomed and to feel as if we belong, despite our communication problems and recall difficulties. By highlighting what remains in dementia, my aim is to encourage society to see people living with dementia with new eyes.

We need communities that welcome people of *all varying physical and cognitive capacities,* where we are accepted within a collective identity. There is no difference between us: I am part of our common existence in the fullness and diversity of humanity. We all have many differences: physical and cognitive ability, looks and many other aspects of our lives, yet we are all part of the richness of human life.

Perspectives on loss of self in dementia have come from outside observers, who can only imagine whether this actually occurs; *they cannot know*. I might forget writing this bit of the book tomorrow, but I will still have unique personal characteristics, which are not lost because of failing cognition. I sense that I continue to exist, moment to moment, relative to my surroundings, and can express this by saying 'I', 'me' and 'my' to locate myself in my psychosocial world. Recognising my continuing sense of being an embodied self within dementia is important for regarding me as having a valid *subjective* perspective, which is my insider's view, giving new insights into the lived experience of dementia.

My sense of being an embodied self, who is sitting here writing this part of my book, is the same embodied self that sat here a moment ago, even if I cannot recall that moment. Many people might find it hard to believe that I could write like this and yet not recall that I sat down to write a day or so ago. But *this is my reality*: a sense of being a continuing embodied self, who I am, then and now, and my damaged brain has not diminished this sense of being present. I still retain a sense of what it means to be Christine.

Many people argue that a loss of sense of self occurs at some time during the lived experience of dementia, and might ask how could I know what might happen much later on in my journey with dementia. However, I have been with people in the later and last stages of dementia, as well as with many others who are living with dementia as best we can. From this viewpoint, we retain a sense of being embodied relational selves, who can continue to find meaningful narratives in the present moment. If people with dementia are assumed to experience a loss of self, we are at risk of less than optimal care, as we are then thought of as being little more than empty shells. I want to turn around these views, so that people with dementia are respected as having a continuing sense of self throughout dementia. *It is a whole person who is being related to and cared for, not some physical presence from which the self has departed.*

I'm still here!

References

Allen, F.B. and Coleman, P.G. (2006) 'Spiritual Perspectives on the Person with Dementia: Identity and Personhood.' In J.C. Hughes, S.J. Louw and S.R. Sabat (eds) *Dementia. Mind, Meaning and Person.* Oxford: Oxford University Press, 205–221.

Alzheimer's Australia (n.d.) *Language Guidelines.* Accessed on 02/03/2018 at www.fightdementia.org.au/files/NATIONAL/documents/language-guidelines-full.pdf.

Alzheimer's Disease International (2000) *Annual Report 1999/2000.* London: Alzheimer's Disease International. Accessed on 02/03/2018 at www.alz.co.uk/adi/pdf/annrep00.pdf.

Ames, S. (2016) 'What happens to the person with dementia?' *Journal of Religion, Spirituality and Aging 28*, 118–135.

Anderson, R.S. (1998) 'On Being Human: The Spiritual Saga of a Creaturely Soul.' In W.S. Brown, N. Murphy and H. Newton Maloney (eds) *Whatever Happened to the Soul? Scientific and Theological Portraits of Human Nature.* Minneapolis, MN: Augsburg Fortress, 175–194.

Aquilina, C. and Hughes, J.C. (2006) 'The Return of the Living Dead: Agency Lost and Found?' In J.C. Hughes, S.J. Louw and S.R. Sabat (eds) *Dementia: Mind, Meaning and Person.* Oxford: Oxford University Press, 143–161.

Augustine (1996) *The Confessions of St. Augustine.* Springdale, PA: Whitaker House.

Baars, J. (2012) 'Critical turns of aging, narrative and time.' *International Journal of Ageing and Later Life 7*, 2, 143–165.

Baker, D.G. (2001) 'Future homemakers and feminist awakenings: Autoethnography as a method in theological education and research.' *Religious Education: The Official Journal of the Religious Education Association 96*, 3, 395–407.

Baldwin, C. and Estey, J. (2015) 'The self and spirituality: Overcoming narrative loss in aging.' *Journal of Religion & Spirituality in Social Work: Social Thought 34*, 2, 205–222.

Brown, W.S. (1998) 'Cognitive Contributions to the Soul.' In W.S. Brown, N. Murphy and H. Newton Maloney (eds) *Whatever Happened to the Soul? Scientific and Theological Portraits of Human Nature.* Minneapolis, MN: Augsburg Fortress, 99–125.

Brown, W.S. (2004) 'Neurological Embodiment of Spirituality and Soul.' In M. Jeeves (ed.) *From Cells to Souls – and Beyond: Changing Portraits of Human Nature.* Grand Rapids, MI: Wm. B. Eerdmans Publishing, 58–76.

Bryan, J. (2016) *Human Being: Insights from Psychology and the Christian Faith.* London: SCM Press.

Bryden, C. (2002) 'A person-centred approach to counselling, psychotherapy and rehabilitation of people diagnosed with dementia in the early stages.' *Dementia 1*, 2, 141–156.

Bryden, C. (2005) *Dancing with Dementia.* London: Jessica Kingsley Publishers.

Bryden, C. (2012) *Who Will I Be When I Die?* (Rev. edn.) London: Jessica Kingsley Publishers.

Bryden, C. (2015a) *Before I Forget.* Melbourne: Penguin Random House Australia.

Bryden, C. (2015b) *Nothing About Us, Without Us.* London: Jessica Kingsley Publishers.

Bryden, C. (2016) 'A spiritual journey into the I–Thou relationship: A personal reflection on living with dementia.' *Journal of Spirituality, Religion and Aging 28*, 1–2, 7–14.

Bryden, C. and MacKinlay, E. (2002) 'Dementia – a Spiritual Journey Towards the Divine: A Personal View of Dementia.' In E. MacKinlay (ed.) *Mental Health and Spirituality in Later Life*. New York, NY: Haworth Pastoral Press, 69–75.

Buber, M. (1937/1970) *I and Thou*, trans. W. Kaufmann. New York, NY: Charles Scribner's Sons.

Churchland, P.S. (2002) 'Self-representation in nervous systems.' *Science 296*, 308–310.

Clandinin, D.J. and Roziek, J. (2006) 'Mapping a Landscape of Narrative Inquiry: Borderland Spaces and Tensions.' In D.J. Clandinin (ed.) *Handbook of Narrative Inquiry: Mapping a Methodology*. Thousand Oaks, CA: Sage, 35–75.

Clark, P.G. (2001) 'Narrative Gerontology in Clinical Practice: Current Applications and Future Prospects.' In G. Kenyon, P. Clark and B. de Vries (eds) *Narrative Gerontology: Theory, Research, and Practice*. New York, NY: Springer Publishing, 193–214.

Crites, S. (1971) 'The narrative quality of experience.' *Journal of the American Academy of Religion 39*, 3, 291–311. Reprinted in S. Hauerwas and L.J. Jones (eds) (1997) *Why Narrative? Readings in Narrative Theology*. Grand Rapids, MI: Wm. B. Eerdmans Publishing, 65–88.

Damasio, A.R. (2010) *Self Comes to Mind*. New York, NY: Pantheon Books.

Denzin, N.K. (2006) 'Analytic autoethnography, or déjà vu all over again.' *Journal of Contemporary Ethnography 35*, 4, 419–428.

Descartes, R. (1637/1912) *A Discourse in Method*, trans. J. Veitch. London: J. M. Dent & Sons.

Doidge, N. (2007) *The Brain That Changes Itself*. Carlton, VI: Scribe Publications.

Ellis, C. and Bochner, A.P. (2000) 'Autoethnography, Personal Narrative, Reflexivity: Researcher as Subject.' In N.K. Denzin and Y.S. Lincoln (eds) *Handbook of Qualitative Research*. New York, NY: Sage, 733–768.

Fiddes, P.S. (2000) 'Story and Possibility: Reflections on the Last Scenes of the Fourth Gospel and Shakespeare's *The Tempest*.' In G. Sauter and J. Barton (eds) *Revelation and Story: Narrative Theology and the Centrality of Story.* Burlington, VT: Ashgate, 29–51.

Frank, A. (2013) *The Wounded Storyteller: Body, Illness and Ethics*, 2nd edn. Chicago, IL: University of Chicago Press.

Green, J.B. (1998) 'Bodies – That Is, Human Lives.' In W.S. Brown, N. Murphy and H. Newton Maloney (eds) *Whatever Happened to the Soul? Scientific and Theological Portraits of Human Nature.* Minneapolis, MN: Augsburg Fortress, 149–173.

Green, J.B. (2008) *Body, Soul, and Human Life (Studies in Theological Interpretation): The Nature of Humanity in the Bible.* Grand Rapids, MI: Baker Academic.

Grenz, S.J. (2006) 'The Social God and the Relational Self: Towards a Theology of the *Imago Dei* in the Postmodern Context.' In R. Lints, M. Horton and M.R. Talbot (eds) *Personal Identity in Theological Perspective.* Grand Rapids, MI: Wm. B. Eerdmans Publishing, 70–93.

Grudzen, M. and Oberle, J.P. (2001) 'Discovering the Spirit in the Rhythm of Time.' In S.H. McFadden and R.C. Atchley (eds) *Ageing and the Meaning of Time: An Interdisciplinary Exploration.* New York, NY: Springer Publishing, 171–188.

Gubrium, J.F. (1986) 'The social preservation of mind: The Alzheimer's disease experience.' *Symbolic Interaction 9*, 1, 37–51.

Hauerwas, S. and Jones, L.J. (1989) *Why Narrative? Readings in Narrative Theology.* Grand Rapids, MI: Wm. B. Eerdmans Publishing.

Holton, R. (2016) 'Memory, persons and dementia.' *Studies in Christian Ethics 29*, 3, 256–260.

Hudson, R.E. (2016) 'God's faithfulness and dementia: Christian theology in context.' *Journal of Religion, Spirituality and Aging 28*, 50–67.

Jones, D.G. (2004) 'The Emergence of Persons.' In M. Jeeves (ed) *From Cells to Souls – and Beyond: Changing Portraits of Human Nature.* Grand Rapids, MI: Wm. B. Eerdmans Publishing, 11–33.

Keck, D. (1996) *Forgetting Whose We Are. Alzheimer's Disease and the Love of God.* Nashville, TN: Abingdon Press.

Kenyon, G.M. and Randall, W. L. (2001) 'Narrative Gerontology: An Overview.' In G. Kenyon, P. Clark and B. de Vries (eds) *Narrative Gerontology: Theory, Research, and Practice.* New York, NY: Springer Publishing, 3–18.

Kevern, P. (2010) 'Alzheimer's and the dementia of God.' *International Journal of Public Theology 4*, 237–253.

Kevern, P. (2012) 'Community without memory? In search of an ecclesiology of liberation in the company of people with dementia.' *International Journal for the Study of the Christian Church 12*, 1, 44–54.

Kinghorn, W.A. (2016) '"I am still with you:" Dementia and the Christian wayfarer.' *Journal of Religion, Spirituality and Aging 28*, 1–2, 98–117.

Kitwood, T. (1997) *Dementia Reconsidered.* Maidenhead: Open University Press.

Kuhl, D.R. and Westwood, M. (2001) 'A Narrative Approach to Integration and Healing among the Terminally Ill.' In G. Kenyon, P. Clark and B. de Vries (eds) *Narrative Gerontology: Theory, Research, and Practice.* New York, NY: Springer Publishing, 311–330.

Locke, J. (1975) *An Essay Concerning Human Understanding*, ed. P.H. Nidditch. Oxford: Clarendon Press.

MacIntyre, A. (1981) 'The Virtues, the Unity of a Human Life and the Concept of a Tradition.' In S. Hauerwas and L.J. Jones (eds) (1989) *Why Narrative? Readings in Narrative Theology.* Grand Rapids, MI: Wm. B. Eerdmans Publishing, 89–110.

MacIntyre, A. (1999) *Dependent Rational Animals.* Peru, IL: Open Court Publishing.

MacKinlay, E. (2011) 'Walking with a Person into Dementia: Creating Care Together.' In A. Jewell (ed) *Spirituality and Personhood in Dementia.* London: Jessica Kingsley Publishers.

MacKinlay, E. (2016) 'Journeys with people who have dementia.' *Journal of Religion, Spirituality and Aging 28*, 24–36.

MacKinlay, E. and Trevitt, C. (2012) *Finding Meaning in the Experience of Dementia: The Place of Spiritual Reminiscence Work.* London: Jessica Kingsley Publishers.

Macmurray, J. (1999) *Persons in Relation.* Amherst, NY: Humanity Books.

Matyushkin, D.P. (2008) 'The hypothesis about neurophysiological basis of the inner self.' *International Journal of Psychophysiology 69,* 283–284.

McFadden, S.H., Ingram, M. and Baldauf, V. (2000) 'Actions, Feelings and Values: Foundations of Meaning and Personhood in Dementia.' In M.A. Kimble (ed) *Viktor Frankl's Contribution to Spirituality and Aging.* New York, NY: Haworth Pastoral Press, 67–86.

Moen, T. (2006) 'Reflections on the narrative research approach.' *International Journal of Qualitative Methods 5,* 4, 56–69.

Murphy, N. (1998) 'Nonreductive Physicalism: Philosophical Issues.' In W.S Brown, N. Murphy and H. Newton Maloney (eds) *Whatever Happened to the Soul? Scientific and Theological Portraits of Human Nature.* Minneapolis, MN: Augsburg Fortress, 127–148.

Murphy, N. (2006) *Bodies and Souls, or Spirited Bodies? (Current Issues in Theology).* New York, NY: Cambridge University Press.

Neibuhr, H.R. (1941) 'The Story of Our Life, the Meaning of Revelation.' In S. Hauerwas and L.J. Jones (eds) (1989) *Why Narrative? Readings in Narrative Theology.* Grand Rapids, MI: Wm. B. Eerdmans Publishing, 21–44.

Polkinghorne, J. (1996) *Beyond Science: The Wider Human Context.* Cambridge: Cambridge University Press.

Poll, J.B. and Smith, T.B. (2003) 'The spiritual self: Toward a conceptualization of spiritual identity development.' *Journal of Psychology and Theology 31,* 2, 129–142.

Post, S.G. (1995) *The Moral Challenge of Alzheimer's Disease.* Baltimore, MD: Johns Hopkins University Press.

Post, S.G. (1998) 'A Moral Case for Nonreductive Physicalism.' In W. S. Brown, N. Murphy and H. Newton Maloney (eds) *Whatever Happened to the Soul? Scientific and Theological Portraits of Human Nature.* Minneapolis, MN: Augsburg Fortress, 195–212.

Post, S.G. (2004) 'Alzheimer's and grace.' *First Things: A Monthly Journal of Religion and Public Life 142*, 12–14.

Post, S.G. (2006) 'Respectare: Moral Respect for the Lives of the Deeply Forgetful.' In J.C. Hughes, S.J. Louw and S.R. Sabat (eds) *Dementia: Mind, Meaning and Person.* Oxford: Oxford University Press, 223–234.

Reinders, H.S. (2008) *Receiving the Gift of Friendship: Profound Disability, Theological Anthropology, and Ethics.* Grand Rapids, MI: Wm. B. Eerdmans Publishing.

Sabat, S.R. (2001) *The Experience of Alzheimer's Disease: Life Through a Tangled Veil.* Oxford: Blackwell.

Sabat, S.R. (2010) 'Stern words on the mind–brain problem: Keeping the whole person in mind.' *New Ideas in Psychology 28*, 2, 168–174.

Sabat, S.R. and Gladstone, C.M. (2010) 'What intact social cognition and social behavior reveal about cognition in the moderate stage of Alzheimer's disease: A case study.' *Dementia 9*, 1, 61–78.

Sabat, S.R., Johnson, A., Swarbrick, C. and Keady, J. (2011) 'The "demented other" or simply "a person"? Extending the philosophical discourse of Naue and Kroll through the situated self.' *Nursing Philosophy 12*, 4, 282–292.

Sabat, S.R. and Lee, J.M. (2011) 'Relatedness among people diagnosed with dementia: Social cognition and the possibility of friendship.' *Dementia 11*, 3, 315–327.

Sacks, O. (1985) *The Man Who Mistook His Wife for a Hat.* London: Picador.

Swinton, J. (2011) 'Being in the Moment. Developing a Contemplative Approach to Spiritual Care with People Who Have Dementia.' In A. Jewell (ed) *Spirituality and Personhood in Dementia.* London: Jessica Kingsley Publishers.

Swinton, J. (2012) *Dementia: Living in the Memories of God.* Grand Rapids, MI: Wm. B. Eerdmans Publishing.

Swinton, J. (2014) 'What's in a name?' *International Journal of Practical Theology 18*, 2, 234–247.

Tillich, P. (1969) *The Courage to Be.* London: Collins.

Vanier, J. (1979) *Community and Growth.* Homebush, Sydney: St Paul Publications.

Wall, S. (2015) 'An autoethnography on learning about autoethnography.' *International Journal of Qualitative Methods 5*, 2, 146–160.

Walton, H. (2002) 'Speaking in signs: Narrative and trauma in pastoral theology.' *Scottish Journal of Healthcare Chaplaincy 5*, 2, 2–5.

Weaver, G.D. (1986) 'Senile dementia and a resurrection theology.' *Theology Today 42*, 4, 444–456.

Wiesel, E. (1992) *The Forgotten*. New York, NY: Schocken.

Wyatt, J. (2009) *Matters of Life and Death: Human Dilemmas in the Light of the Christian Faith*. Nottingham: Intervarsity Press.

Zizoulas, J.D. (1975) 'Human capacity and human incapacity: A theological exploration of personhood.' *Scottish Journal of Theology 28*, 5, 401–444.

Index